The ALZHEIMER'S
SOLUTION

MORE PRAISE FOR *THE ALZHEIMER'S SOLUTION*

"This provocative book is a must read for anyone interested in biology and aging. The authors have crafted a brilliant document with both practical and theoretical implications for how we age."

Bruce L. Miller, MD
A. W. Clausen Distinguished Professor of Neurology
and director of the Memory & Aging Center,
University of California, San Francisco

"In *The Alzheimer's Solution*, Kosik and Clegg take a fresh look at how dementia is addressed in the United States. Combining scientific and medical insight with a gift for clear expression, they show how society's resources might be better used to give more humane and appropriate care. This book is necessary reading for students, concerned family members, and policymakers."

Sam Wang
Associate professor of neuroscience,
Princeton University, and author of
*Welcome to Your Brain: Why You Lose Your
Car Keys but Never Forget How to Drive*

KENNETH S. KOSIK, MD, *and* ELLEN CLEGG

The ALZHEIMER'S
SOLUTION

How Today's Care Is Failing Millions
and How We Can Do Better

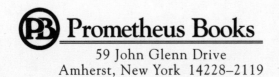
59 John Glenn Drive
Amherst, New York 14228–2119

Published 2010 by Prometheus Books

Inquiries should be addressed to
Prometheus Books
59 John Glenn Drive
Amherst, New York 14228–2119
VOICE: 716–691–0133
FAX: 716–691–0137
WWW.PROMETHEUSBOOKS.COM

14 13 12 11 10   5 4 3 2 1

Library of Congress Cataloging-in-Publication Data

Kosik, K. S. (Kenneth S.), 1950–
    The Alzheimer's solution : how today's care is failing millions—and how we can do better / by Kenneth S. Kosik and Ellen Clegg.
        p. ; cm.
    Includes bibliographical references and index.
    ISBN 978–1–61614–208–7 (pbk. : alk. paper)
    1. Alzheimer's disease—United States. I. Clegg, Ellen, 1950– II. Title.
    [DNLM: 1. Alzheimer's Disease—United States. 2. Aged—United States.
3. Health Policy—United States. 4. Health Services for the Aged—United States.
5. Quality of Health Care—United States. WT 155 K86a 2010]

RC523.K67 2010
362.196'831—dc22   2009019524

Printed in the United States of America on acid-free paper

CONTENTS

ACKNOWLEDGMENTS

We owe a great deal of gratitude to those who helped in so many ways—some with their comments and insights, others with their patience—as we invested the long hours to bring this book to fruition. They are Miyoung Chun; three generations of Kosik family—Selma, Abe, Leah, Russell, Sabrina, and Eena; Tom and Eli Harriman; Hether Briggs; Bradley Joseph; John LaPuma; Dennis Baker; Robert Harbaugh; Paul Erikson; Matt Tirrell; Martin Moskowitz; Bill Mowry, Nancy Brown, Michelle Woodhouse, Mike Gazzaniga; William Grant; June Kinoshita; Francisco Lopera; the many families in Colombia who suffer from familial Alzheimer's disease; and Julie Lawson and all the members of her extended family. Thanks to our agent, Janice Pieroni, a tireless advocate, and to our publicist, Gail Leondar-Wright. Thanks, of course, to Ellen Zucker, Judy Zucker, Jonathan Gagen, Jake Zucker, Doris Clegg, Barry Clegg and Roberta Swanson, Dennis Clegg and Terri Burgess, and Michelle Cerulli. Special thanks to Lisa Tuite, *Boston Globe* librarian, for her research support and warm advice on all manner of projects.

PREFACE

Sometimes we must travel far away to see ourselves more accurately, to see what we have and what we lack. And so in the course of my research on Alzheimer's disease, I traveled to the state of Antioquia in Colombia and saw the reflection of our challenge in facing this disease among the campesinos of a remote community. Here, a rare genetic form of Alzheimer's disease that strikes in middle age takes an enormous toll on families and communities. Colombia is not the solution to what ails Alzheimer's disease care in the United States, but the story wakes us up to some of the missing pieces in our care model. In the absence of a sophisticated medical system in these rural areas, families must care for those with dementia on their own; they must continue to integrate them into their lives rather than creating the isolation centers we call assisted living facilities or nursing homes. Children are not excluded from witnessing the final chapter of life. Sometimes our goal seems simply to make those with dementia invisible in our daily lives.

The plight of dementia has moved us to build a research empire and a care industry whose costs represent a significant fraction of the healthcare quagmire we now face. Like most large, amorphous social structures assembled over time, what we have is a patchwork laden with historical baggage and outdated views that is unprepared for the magnitude of the problem. Alzheimer's disease gets shoehorned into a medical system that has no place for it. As currently configured, the disease fits neither into a tertiary care center, where the economic engine is surgery, nor into the primary-care practice, where the expertise in topics from diet to genetics is missing, as are the breadth of nonmedical services and the economic incentives. Physicians are limited to what is amenable to pills or the knife. Alzheimer's disease is not amenable to either. It is our strong conviction that we as a society can do a far better job—and do so more effectively and at a lower cost.

Step one is detecting Alzheimer's disease in the brain before a person becomes impaired. The tools of early detection—genetic predictions, biomarker testing, and brain imaging—are in hand. These tools take us beyond prevention programs that simply exhort the watchwords to anyone who will listen. The modern tools of early detection allow personalized risk assessment and personalized approaches to an intervention program.

While the medical profession all but ignores the problem of dementia, the gap is filled by fringe elements, such as health products and vitamin vendors, and Web sites filled with dubious information and blinking advertisements. It is perhaps an irony of our time that with so many avenues to knowledge at our command, we can find ourselves starved for information in a sea churning with nothing but information. The particular knowledge craved, for example, by those given a life-threatening diagnosis, often lies outside the expertise of physicians—even specialists. While flickers of hope appear on the Web through encounters and a shared experience with others, judging the reliability of this experience—and its fit with our own—can be difficult. Nevertheless, the means is there in the vast reach of the Internet to find information and test its reliability. No longer is one person—an expert—expected to know everything and render infallible judgment. That burdensome view of the expert physician is no longer tenable, nor is it necessary.

Our goal is to treat Alzheimer's disease before it occurs. We now have good evidence for a set of preventive measures that, if adopted, can delay the onset of the disease to the point that competing mortality will markedly reduce its incidence. Delaying the onset of dementia by five years would halve the prevalence of dementia. The reduction in costs and suffering of early intervention would be enormous.

Most of the interventions are well known and the data that support them are overwhelming. They include exercise, attention to diet, cognitive stimulation, social engagement, and control of diabetes, blood pressure, and lipid levels. But, as the all-too-familiar saying goes, the devil is in the details. How much exercise, which diet, and what exactly *is* cognitive stimulation? How can we encourage adherence to a program that offers what people need, what they want, and what they can do?

And social engagement is not for everybody. We need to consider that guidelines are designed for populations, but that we are a community of individuals.

Alzheimer's is one of the few serious diseases that run their course without physical pain. Of course an Alzheimer patient can experience pain, but the disease itself is not painful. Needless to say, the painlessness of Alzheimer's disease offers little comfort. Why? Because Alzheimer's disease robs us of something more valuable than a limb or sight or mobility. It robs us of our own identities—first our memories and personality, and then our dignity. Alzheimer's disease steals our faculties little by little. We never really know how much of the world the Alzheimer patient can grasp. The challenge of understanding the feelings of others is vast under the best of conditions, but in the case of Alzheimer's disease we must glean meaning from a transient facial expression or an eye movement. Sometimes, inside that enigmatic look of an Alzheimer patient may lie a hope, even a request, to bring an otherwise wonderful life to a dignified conclusion.

1

THE INSPIRATION

I looked down the dark road along which the bikers would begin their trek the next morning. A few streetlights trailed off in the distance, and then the road went dark. It made me think of the road the Alzheimer patient travels. For us, at nightfall the ride stops, and we rejuvenate ourselves in the soft, incandescent glow of lanterns and the circle of tent light and the comfort of friends. But for the Alzheimer patient, the road just keeps going, on into the darkness.
—KENNETH S. KOSIK, FROM A PUBLIC PRESENTATION
AT THE MEMORY RIDE, BOSTON

THE LARGEST KINDRED IN THE WORLD
WITH FAMILIAL ALZHEIMER'S DISEASE

Faviola's extended family is gathered in her living room. They live in Pedregal, a small barrio near Medellín in Colombia. In the clean but spare house, far from the nearest clinic, we are performing a neurological exam on her husband, Ramón, who, despite his Alzheimer's disease, does a reasonable job of caring for himself. "With your forefinger, touch my finger and then touch your nose," says Dr. Francisco Lopera, who demonstrates the task. In 1987 Dr. Lopera, a prominent neurologist in Medellín and professor at the University of Antioquia School of Medicine, and some of his colleagues discovered the largest extended family in the world with familial Alzheimer's disease. Faviola and Ramón are members of this extended family.

As a young associate professor at Harvard Medical School, I met Dr.

Lopera in 1992 while on a trip to Bogotá, Colombia, where I was working with the Colombian neurosurgeon Enrique Osorio to help develop neuroscience research in his country. After a lecture I gave on Alzheimer's disease, Dr. Lopera introduced himself and told me about several large families in his home state of Antioquia. Many members of these families had typical Alzheimer's disease, but its onset was unusually early, often in the late forties. As his story unfolded, it became increasingly clear that in the valley on the outskirts of the state's capital, Medellín, and in the countryside beyond, a mysterious form of Alzheimer's disease was quietly claiming the lives of its inhabitants. As can happen only at a stage of life when very little prevents us from following our instincts and the allure of the unknown, the next morning I boarded a plane from Bogotá to Medellín. Thus began a fifteen-year ongoing collaboration.

Many years and many trips to Colombia later, after many scientific papers with Dr. Lopera, I return to Colombia and visit the small town of Pedregal, about an hour's drive from Medellín. Faviola, in her early forties, and Ramón, in his late forties, belong to one branch of an enormous extended family. On each of my many visits to Colombia, I am impressed anew at how a remote and isolated culture suffering from Alzheimer's disease has adapted to the tragedy of dementia. What has become quite clear to me is that here in the United States we can learn something about caring for Alzheimer's disease from these families.[1]

"With your forefinger, touch my finger and then touch your nose," repeats Dr. Lopera. Ramón extends his arm and touches Dr. Lopera's nose, not his own. The two younger children watching the spectacle giggle: "Papi touched the doctor's nose!" They are Ramón's eleven-year-old son, Alonso, and his ten-year-old niece, Solana. The third child, his thirteen-year-old daughter, Luz Marina, does not giggle. She has crossed some boundary, one that marks an individual's awareness of the finitude of life, and watches solemnly.

Next Dr. Lopera tests Ramón with other instructions while he demonstrates each command: clap your hands, whistle, imitate how you would comb your hair, brush your teeth. Ramón's expression is helpless and puzzled; he is frustrated by his inability to comply with the instructions of the respected doctor. Dr. Lopera asks him if he can hop on one foot, and demonstrates. Success. Ramón begins to hop on one foot. He hops around the living room, but does not understand when asked to stop hopping. Like an overwound toy, he hops out to the kitchen and back around the couch and between the circle of chairs and looks to Dr. Lopera for some sign of approval. The two younger children's giggles turn to outright laughter. The thirteen-year-old is silent.

When the exam is complete we re-form our circle and chat with Faviola and her two sisters, Altagracia and Beatrice. Ramón's niece sits on his lap, her head leaning against his chest, and his son sits proudly next to his dad. All three kids look adoringly at their dad—he is one of their best playmates, endlessly patient with the repetitive games that engross youngsters. They all cling to him as if their grasp could somehow prevent him from slipping away. Confidence in the constancy of the moment-to-moment present has been shaken here as each new failure, each minuscule decline, marks Ramón's fade from his family.

Faviola tells us how she and her husband moved about ten years ago from a pueblo called Angostora, several hours away from Medellín, to the outskirts of the big city, where they opened a *tienda* or small neighborhood grocery store. To get to Pedregal one has to navigate the traffic-choked streets from the well-heeled Poblado sector, with its lively nightlife and outdoor restaurants, through the grimy outbound routes where street vendors dodge the traffic with their wares. Here the streets are lined with modest, well-kept two-story homes and corner grocery stores. About two years ago Ramón began to repeat himself in conversation. He might tell his wife some news about a cousin back in Angostora, and only ten or twenty minutes later he would repeat the news as if he were telling her for the first time. Faviola had seen this problem before. Her mother had also developed Alzheimer's disease.

Just out of sight from where we sit is a small room furnished with only a bed. Under the starched white sheet Faviola's sixty-three-year-old mother, Mercedes, lies silent and crooked and motionless, except for the slow rise and fall of her breathing. She has had Alzheimer's disease for twelve years. She does not respond when Dr. Lopera calls her name, even when he leans over and says her name directly in her ear. He lifts her arm and gently tries to extend her forearm, but it remains rigid and flexed at the elbow. He tries to extend her knee or flex her neck—she is rigid everywhere. Sometimes she grimaces at these passive attempts at movement. She is stuck in the final round of a bizarre game of freeze tag, touched by a creeping death that has claimed more and more of her body after taking her mind years ago.

On the way toward this fate, mobility can come to a halt in piece-meal fashion. Not long before this trip, in a nursing home back in the States, I saw a man whose neck was permanently bent forward, his chin close to his chest, leaving nothing more than his own dressing gown in his visual field as he shuffled his feet to power his wheelchair up and down the corridor, the nursing staff clearing the path. Often the muscles of facial expression become frozen. I saw another man in the same nursing home who was still able to walk, but whose face was frozen in an expression of permanent horror. Whether sitting in front of his own birthday cake surrounded by family or settling into a freshly made bed, his face registered shock and fear, as if his children had just been murdered before his eyes. This single fixed look was all that remained of a once vast repertoire of facial expressions and their corresponding emotions, all now drained away.

While Dr. Lopera examines Mercedes, the children scamper in and out of the room. They hold their grandma's unresponsive hand as the adults talk around the bed. Over and over again in Colombia one sees the children fully involved with the affected members of their families, no matter how debilitated. In a culture that has no retirement communities, nursing homes, and hospice, those with Alzheimer's disease are not cordoned off, are not made invisible. There is not the timidity or fear of elders whose health is failing, who are wrinkled, arthritic, and bent over. Elders are not removed from their families, and so the entire life span has continuity. Children see and live daily with what could await them—a fate that may not be pleasant, but neither is it shrouded in the faux good humor of hired staff in assisted living facilities tending room after room of patients who have become depersonalized objects. Without even the possibility of moving loved ones to an institution where they might spend their final days among strangers, the long, slow transition to death unfolds in the home.

When we return to the living room, Faviola tells us that the eldest of her twelve siblings, now forty-eight years old, is beginning to show the earliest signs of Alzheimer's disease. Her eyes are bright and engaging and filled with resilience as she relates this family history. Her quieter sister, Altagracia, nods and sometimes fills in details. They have watched their mother deteriorate, and now, as their generation approaches midlife, the disease is again making its inexorable appearance.

This is familial Alzheimer's disease, a rare, inherited form of the disease that differs from the more common variety only in its early age of onset. Less than 1 percent of all Alzheimer's disease is caused solely by a genetic mutation. The remaining 99 percent of cases, called sporadic, have no known cause, although genetics do have a modest influence over sporadic Alzheimer's disease. The greatest single risk for Alzheimer's disease is advancing age, but familial Alzheimer's disease typically has its onset in middle age. The young age of onset is most distressing in several families I have seen in Colombia in which an elderly grandma—whose husband died of Alzheimer's disease many years earlier, perhaps in his fifties—is now caring for three or more of her children, all of whom also have Alzheimer's disease. Often the small children of these Alzheimer victims also live in the same house.

The onset of Alzheimer's disease in midlife has created some particularly poignant situations. Consuela, now in her seventies, is a prime example. Many years ago the families of Angostora, where she was born, celebrated one of the saints' days with a fiesta that carried on into the evening. That night she met her future husband—the two of them talked until the sun came up. She was nineteen and he was twenty-three. Like many people from the countryside, she and her new husband, Octavio, moved closer to the big city of Medellín in the hope of carving out a better life. They lived in the outskirts of the city, along the railroad tracks in the last house on a lane that trailed off into a field. There, over the next two decades, the couple had thirteen children. Ten years after the last child was born, Octavio lay moribund in a nearly empty room of their simple home. Shortly after the birth of the youngest child, he had begun to repeat himself, to the annoyance of the family. A few months later he had outbursts of anger at his wife because he believed she was having numerous affairs with the neighbors. Reasoning with him about the impossibility of his misconceptions only angered him more. Sometimes he threatened to kill her.

Consuela said that what was most difficult was the sameness, day after day. She remembered how she used to look forward to Sunday, the one day of the week when her husband and older children did not go off to work in the coffee plantations. She especially looked forward to December, when people outline the streets of the entire neighborhood with candles and celebrate the wonderful Colombian custom Novena, a nine-day period when each evening neighbors visit each other, exchange gifts, and gather outside to sing *villancicos*, or Christmas carols. Now, every day was the same—Octavio did not know one day from the other, and every day he asked the same questions and displayed the same anger. There was no reprieve, no holidays, no difference between the morning and the night. After nearly eight years of this suffering, Octavio grew quiet and apathetic. His body and face became rigid. Each day Consuela moved him to a chair where he sat immobile, without looking or reacting to anything around him. Then the time came when she could no longer move him to his chair and he remained in bed. He lay beneath the immaculate white sheets, neatly tucked in at each corner, his head tilted to the side in an odd position, his eyes neither quite closed nor quite open. Except for the iron bed and a crucifix hanging on the wall over his head, the room was profoundly empty, even of sound. It was a living tomb that enshrined his memory while he still breathed, but did little else. It was the dress rehearsal for eternity. For several years Octavio remained in this condition, and all that time he never developed a single bedsore; he never appeared soiled.

Seventeen years after her husband's death, when Consuela was sixty-three years old, her eldest child began to repeat himself. Another decade passed, and now the seventy-three-year-old Consuela cares for two sons and one daughter. The eldest son, now fifty-four years old, lies moribund in the same room, in the same bed as his father. Another son, in his late forties, roams the house at odd hours and sometimes threatens his mother because he thinks she is flirting with a neighbor. Consuela's daughter, also in her midforties, sits silently in a chair all day. Some of Consuela's grandchildren, now deprived of a parent, also live in the house.

The oldest of the grandchildren, now in their early twenties, do not want to know anything about this insidious gene that has tracked the generations of their family. When we asked twenty-year-old Maricela, whose mother spends her days sitting in a chair, about her future, she was confident that she would escape the scourge. She was obviously uncomfortable with the topic and a bit annoyed by the questions. But sometimes I met children of a similar age in other families with the disease who felt certain they would get the disease. I asked one young man why he was so convinced he would get the same condition as his father. The boy said to me, "Because I look like my father." Some notions about inheritance were beginning to inform their views, but their opinions were often flawed by imperfect knowledge of how traits genetically segregate. There is no reason to believe, for example, that the many genes that control an individual's physical appearance are in any way related to the gene responsible for familial Alzheimer's disease.

In Faviola's family something else is amiss. Not only is the mutant gene present in her own blood relatives, but she has married into a family that also carries the mutant gene. This enormous genetic burden stacks the deck against her children. With their dad affected by the Alzheimer mutation, those children sitting next to him have a 50 percent chance of inheriting his disease gene. At first glance, their chances are a simple flip of a coin. But this family cluster is unusual even among the larger extended family, because Faviola's mother also has the mutant gene. If Faviola has also inherited the mutant gene, then her children would be offspring of parents who both carry the Alzheimer gene, and their odds of getting the disease soar to 75 percent.[2]

In our research team's genetic work with Lopera, along with another collaborator, Alison Goate at Washington University in St. Louis, in

1995 we found the mutant gene that affects Ramón and Faviola's extended family. To reach this goal, the many branches of the family and their complex relationships had to be drawn accurately. Finding the gene depended on getting accurate information about the inheritance pattern of the disease. If we mistakenly assigned a child who eventually developed Alzheimer's disease to the wrong parent, the genetic data would be flawed. For example, paternity might be in question because the father died and the mother remarried when the child was very young. Collecting family histories and getting accurate information required numerous visits to the remote villages where the families lived. This laborious task was painstakingly carried out over years by Lopera and the project nurse, Lucia Madrigal. The common practice in Antioquia of having twelve to fifteen children ballooned the family trees. Because the people often remain within their small villages, the frequency of consanguineous marriage—that is, the practice of marrying one's cousin—is high. For all these reasons, drawing the family trees was a challenge—names and family relationships brimmed over the edges of large sheets of paper and existing family tree software was often overtaxed by the tangled web of relationships. Still the families grew.

Twelve large families with the same rare mutation were eventually identified. Because the mutation is so rare, it could not have arisen in all these families by chance. The twelve families had to be related to each other, even though the family members themselves had lost track of any connection. By searching church records and reconstructing their ancestries, Lopera filled in deeper family histories that ultimately connected the twelve families near the time many of the small Antioquian towns were founded in the 1700s. Today, well over five thousand individuals populate the extended family tree. They are, by far, the largest family in the world to harbor a mutation that inevitably leads to Alzheimer's disease, and they contributed to the discovery of this very important Alzheimer gene. Those with the mutation will get the disease with nearly 100 percent certainty once they reach their fourth or fifth decade. The average age of onset is forty-eight years old.

How does this work on a genomic level? What we call the Alzheimer gene is a mutant form of a gene that we all have. The gene is called presenilin and can harbor mutations that cause Alzheimer's disease. The gene is, in fact, essential for life; without it, a person cannot survive past birth. Even though the gene is critical for life, its existence was not suspected before it showed up in familial Alzheimer's disease. People with a mistake or mutation in the presenilin gene can survive because the mutant form of the gene is compatible with life, but they develop Alzheimer's disease later in life. Although we were hot on the trail of the gene, it was Peter St. George-Hyslop—working with another large family in Calabria, Italy—who got there first.[3] Having found the gene, he earned the right to name it. He dubbed it presenilin because it causes a "presenile dementia," or early onset dementia. Mutations like the one in Antioquia and a slightly different mutation in the same gene in Calabria are called private mutations because each is found in a single family. A small difference in the location of the mutation allows us to distinguish the Antioquian from the Calabrian family. In contrast, genetic mutations such as the one that causes sickle cell anemia are present in many families and are therefore more widely distributed.

After the discovery of the Alzheimer mutations, other scientists found that if the gene is removed from a mouse, the mouse dies around the time of birth. These experiments and others showed that the gene plays a critical role in the embryonic development of many organisms, including humans. Presenilin is part of a protein complex that works as an enzyme to cut another protein, which in turn controls the transition of an embryonic cell to a mature cell. Ironically, this protein that is so critical to development at the very beginning of life becomes a culprit in degeneration late in life. The process of evolution selects for traits over time that help us survive long enough so that we can reproduce and pass our genes along to offspring. As we age past that point, however, mutations in genes that had no effect on our ability to bear children and remain silent for decades can begin to damage our bodies. No one knows why people who carry the presenilin mutation from the time of conception show no ill effects of the mutation until many years later when Alzheimer disease strikes.

Like all of our approximately twenty-five thousand genes, the presenilin gene consists of a long series of the four different nucleotides that correspond to the letters A, T, G, and C. These letters represent the building blocks of the genetic code. They are used over and over again—nearly one hundred thousand times—to make the presenilin gene. When one of these letters is mutated—say, an A to C—at a position where the gene uses that letter to encode an amino acid (the building blocks of proteins), the individual with this single mistake will develop Alzheimer's disease as an adult.

Because mutations can have grave consequences, nature has developed several protection systems to prevent mutations. First, mutations are rare; usually our genomes replicate themselves from generation to generation without errors. However, errors occasionally slip through the protection net. Of our three billion nucleotides, only errors in very few positions make a difference. When a mistake arises in a neutral position, it is passed on to future generations but usually remains unnoticed. These benign changes are called *polymorphisms* (see chapter 3 for more details). Much less commonly, a person has an error in the genome that does permit survival into the childbearing years but the person is unable to have children and the mutation is lost when that person dies. Even more rarely, a mutation is beneficial in a way that those with the mutation have more surviving progeny; in these cases the mutation eventually becomes more prevalent in the population. What began as an error in the genome is transformed into a useful trait. One of the best-known examples is the lactase gene, which allows most of us (unless the gene carries a mutation) to digest the lactose in milk. This gene arose through a beneficial mutation around the time when humans domesticated cattle and conferred a survival advantage on those able to drink cow's milk.

These random mistakes in copying our genes over generations—and whether the mistakes are good, bad, or indifferent to our survival—are the engine of evolution. In the complex play between random mutations and fitness, a single error with sad consequences destined to reverberate down through many generations happened to occur in an ancestor of Faviola. This mutation, however, did not fit so neatly into any of the usual categories. On the one hand, those with the mutation suffer from a disease that compromises their survival, but because the disease does not have its onset until after childbearing age, it is not easily eliminated.

Where did this mutation come from, and why has it assumed such gravity in the community? There had to be an original founder, the person in whom the mutation first arose. Who was this person? We know from the distance the gene has spread—well beyond third- and fourth-degree cousins—that the founder dates back close to the time when Spanish conquistadores first came to Colombia, or even earlier. This measure of genetic spread can be understood by this simple example: if two cousins both have the mutation, then the gene has to have arisen within the generation of their grandparents or earlier, because the cousins have different parents.

A Brief History of the Region

The population of Antioquia today is a patchwork of peoples stemming from a rich history of migration and conquest. Mariscal Jorge Robledo is called "el conquistador de Antioquia." He founded the first of the Spanish towns in Antioquia—Cartago in 1540 and the original capital, Santa Fe de Antioquia, in 1541. Antioquia is a state in modern-day Colombia, but at the time of these conquistadors it was part of the Nuevo Reino de Granada (New Kingdom of Granada). The heartland of this region is the Aburrá Valley, a natural basin of the Medellín River located on the Central Range of the Andes, between the Magdalen and Cauca valleys. Historically, the region, located between two mountain chains, was nearly inaccessible. Just before the arrival of the Spanish and accelerating after their arrival, Amerindian populations were decimated. European diseases and cruel conditions ravaged their population. In the Aburrá Valley, few, if any, living traces of the indigenous people remain. The Spanish also fought among themselves, mostly over land rights and authority. Robledo himself was choked and beheaded, condemned to death in 1546 by Sebastián de Belalcázar, one of the more ruthless characters of the time. By the seventeenth and eighteenth centuries, Basque families from the North of Spain joined earlier settlers in the Aburrá Valley in and around Medellín.

The people of this region call themselves Paisa. Paisa see themselves as different from the rest of the Colombian population and often like to speculate about their origins. Perhaps they are Basque; perhaps Sephardic *marranos*, the Spanish Jews who were forced to convert to Catholicism during the Spanish Inquisition; perhaps Africans or Iberians from Extremadura who came in the sixteenth century or from Andalucía who came in the seventeenth century. Some of the towns founded by the early settlers, such as the picturesque village El Retiro, have families with the Alzheimer mutation today. Somewhere among the people of this chaotic historical transition the Alzheimer mutation was harbored, perhaps without even a trace of Alzheimer's disease because life expectancy was so short.

Just after a mutation occurs, its persistence is a matter of chance, and its chance to be passed on to the next generation can be slim. If the owner of the mutation dies without having children or if his or her children do not inherit the mutation, that mutation is lost—the mutant gene goes extinct. One can imagine that in the dense vegetation of the Colombian sierras and in the villages where violence has flared over many decades, those few early individuals with the mutation survived against the odds of high mortality. The fragile links of the early inheritance chain continued unbroken as a result of hundreds of chance events; many chance factors conspired in order for the mutation to gain the prevalence it has today. In genetics this phenomenon is called *genetic drift*, and it accounts for a great deal of the genetic variety we observe among human populations.

What has become clear from modern genetic studies by Andres Ruiz, a geneticist from Colombia who now lives in London, is that the

Paisa ancestry consists mainly of Iberian men and Amerindian women who were a diverse mix of tribes grouped under the Chibchan language group. The genomes of Paisa today are an admixture, or blending, of these two ancestries. The male history is marked upon the Y chromosome, which is present only in males and carries the genetic history of one's male ancestry. Another stretch of DNA, in a part of the cell called the *mitochondrion*, carries the genetic history of female ancestry. Over many generations, people living on the Iberian Peninsula accumulated some innocuous genetic errors—polymorphisms—that were passed down to subsequent generations precisely because they were innocuous, and so there was no pressure to rid the genome of them. The Amerindians also have their own polymorphisms. What is revealing is that the Paisa have polymorphisms from the Iberian peninsula on their Y chromosome and Amerindian polymorphisms in their mitochondrial DNA. The story is all too clear. Among the conquests of the invaders were the Amerindian women, and their offspring became the Paisa. Amerindian men and Iberian women made insignificant genetic contributions to the current population. In this way, the human genome can reveal the history of a people.

The Dilemma of Predictive Genetic Testing

What is now rapidly changing for families in Antioquia and elsewhere is the ability of technology to peek backward through an individual's genome at a murky past, stripped of romance or rape, left only with a genetic shadow of generations of matings and procreation. Blood samples taken from Faviola and her oldest daughter, Josefina, age twenty, have also been tested, and the results—whether or not they have the mutant gene—are kept in strict confidence in the Lopera laboratory. Because of the volatility of genetic information, even family members have agreed not to seek access to the information, since genetic counseling services are not available. The decision not to reveal any results of the genetic testing has been an agonizing one and is likely to change as more education and guidance becomes available in the community. All the guidelines for predictive genetic testing require some input from a genetic counselor, and these services are not currently available in Colombia. Clearly this form of genetic paternalism is not a long-term solution to the power genetic information offers. Even now, knowledge of a mutation in the family might convince an at-risk mother to have fewer children. On the other hand, the number of offspring in this community is declining, for unknown reasons, without that incentive.

There is a danger that friends and family, knowing that an individual has the Alzheimer gene, will stigmatize that person even before any symptoms appear. In some of the villages where the mutation is rampant, those affected are called *bobo*, which means "stupid." Genetic counselors and ethicists insist that having a genetic mutation is not the same as having the disease caused by the mutation. Even in the presence of an Alzheimer's genetic mutation, an individual is not considered to have Alzheimer's disease until there are symptoms present. However, carrying a mutation means living with the constant fear that any minor act of forgetfulness—something that all of us do, like misplacing car keys—is the opening shot of the disease. And every such failure might be pounced upon by friends and family as evidence that the disease is imminent.

Perhaps it is best to keep in mind here, the fundamental medical dictum *Primum non nocere*, or "First, do no harm." Both telling and not telling can be harmful, but telling is an active step that can lead to severe depression and even suicide, whereas not telling is a passive act that keeps the physician from actively contributing to a possible bad outcome. Faviola cares for a husband and a mother who both have Alzheimer's disease while living in the shadow of her own genetic inheritance and is watching her children grow up, all the time wondering if this cruel gene will surface yet again among them. Perhaps the dilemma of predictive testing has been most agonizing in the case of Faviola's sister, Altagracia. A strikingly beautiful woman in her thirties—more sophisticated than many about the disease—she has opted for a single life, reluctant to marry and have children because of the possibility that she could pass on the Alzheimer gene. Knowledge of her genetic inheritance might free her of the lock she keeps on her future. Among these families there already exists a rich experience of grappling with a genetic burden. In the United States the growing availability of genetic tests that attempt to predict our future medical conditions has created quandaries for many who might benefit from the experience of the Antioquian families.

From Family Trees to Social Networks

Gazing at family trees, marked with circles for females and squares for males, connected by horizontal lines for couples and vertical lines for their offspring, one watches the generations stroll by, like people-watching at an outdoor café, each passing figure with just a snippet of information from which to infer an individual's life story. Each square and circle on a family tree is a life story. One cannot help speculating how couples met and married, the trials and joys of their child-rearing years, and the circumstances of their deaths. Sometimes, a square or circle yields no vertical line, no offspring, and in these cases their genetic bounty goes extinct. If one of these individuals happened to have a mutation that gave us immunity to Alzheimer's disease, it would be lost.

The family tree is a natural social network in which individuals are bonded through family relationships and more distant relationships are often more socially remote. Having a strong social network—in other words, having many friends—is strongly predictive of the ability to maintain health and well-being in old age. In Colombia, the large families are a natural buffer against the stress of isolation. Caretaker burden is better distributed and information is disseminated. The Colombian experience draws upon the collective power of a social network that is highly applicable to the medical profession. Smaller families may not have a network of people to cushion their needs and so stress levels rise. Shrinking family units leave people vulnerable to the loss of a spouse and subsequent isolation. However, the rapid growth of Internet-based social networking and other community-based networks of caretakers is a potential remedy that we will explore in later chapters.

The idea that social integration can protect health has its scientific roots in the work Lisa Berkman did while a graduate student at the University of California, Berkeley in the 1970s. While poverty strongly contributes to poor health, poverty is not the only sociological factor that affects health. In a comparison of San Francisco neighborhoods, Berkman found that the poor, working-class communities of North Beach and Chinatown—immigrant communities with strong social ties—were far healthier than the many social isolates in the Tenderloin district. The Antioquian families have powerful social links, and these links extend to the broader communities of their towns. The health issues related to Alzheimer's disease are particularly responsive to social networks because so much of the caretaker burden is on the family; when the family is small and isolated, that burden often becomes unbearable.

What has helped connect the large and complex family structures in Colombia is a house called Casa Neurosciencias, near the main hospital in Medellín, Hospital Universitario San Vincente de Paúl. Here, an extended family of up to thirty or forty people can spend the day after a long trip in from the countryside. An open space has comfortable seating and a few tables to unwrap the *empanadas* and *arrepas* brought along for the daylong stay. In another portion of the same open space the doctors and staff congregate so that the professional staff and the families have easy and ready access to each other over the course of a day. Exam rooms and offices border the open area for more private consultation with the patients. All the neuropsychological exams for those in need of testing can be conducted, blood can be drawn, and radiological tests can be obtained across the street in the hospital and reviewed by the team. What is special about the setting is simply the opportunity to spend most of an entire day with a dedicated staff concerned about the many facets of the problems faced by the families and the chance for all the relevant parties—family members, support personnel, and doctors—to delve into the individual and collective problems in a way that cannot be accomplished in strict twenty-minute appointments. Compared to the highly fragmented way in which doctors in the United States see patients—one at a time, with multiple appointments for each test or service—spending a day with an entire extended family is satisfying for everyone. The approach, which brings together all services and caretakers and family in one setting, is also cost effective.

ONE FAMILY'S STORY OF FAMILIAL ALZHEIMER'S: THE NOONANS

Familial Alzheimer's, which strikes early, is not only tragic; it also poses extra challenges for family members, who must struggle with the knowledge that they may carry the very genetic mutation that has struck down a sibling or parent. The disease hits while they are still relatively vital; finding a nursing home to accept someone who is not a frail elder, but can be strong and possibly violent, is a particular challenge. While Julie Noonan Lawson's family has a seemingly rare run of bad luck with early onset Alzheimer's, her situation strikes universal tones, applicable to anyone trying to make sense of the healthcare bureaucracy and meet the needs of a loved one while maintaining some semblance of a normal family life. Although Lawson may be unusual in her political activism, she is typical of any dedicated family member who is determined to find the best care possible, even if it means long nights of research on the Internet and many hours touring inadequate nursing home facilities.

Growing up in Stoughton, Massachusetts, Julie Noonan learned early just how much Alzheimer's could steal from a family. She was three or four years old, finding her way in a tightly knit Irish-American clan in a small town thirty miles from Boston, when her mother began her own hard season of change that would end in institutionalization and early death.

Sitting in her sun-splashed kitchen on a crisp fall afternoon on Cape Cod, Julie—now Julie Noonan Lawson—has an adult's perspective and a lifetime of hard-won medical knowledge. But in 1963, when her mother, Julia Tatro Noonan, began to show mood changes, she was a small girl in a family that was struggling to understand.

"Initially, it was mood more than anything else," Julie says. "She was in her late thirties when she began a kind of personality change. Healthcare professionals saw my mom as being depressed. I mean, she had a lot of kids, so they thought maybe it was postpartum depression, even back then."

As a mother, Julia Tatro Noonan was a twentieth-century Irish American archetype, and the Noonan family's particular trajectory has been replicated any number of times and braided into the colorful fabric of Boston. Julia coordinated the daily lives of ten children, cooking meals, tending to homework, and doing laundry while her husband, John, worked as a firefighter. When Julia began to forget, the daily life of the house began to spin apart. Worst of all, her daughter remembers, the ample generosity and love that kept the Noonans together began to fray.

Julia received shock treatments—a stock therapy of the day—but her depression did not seem to lift. Doctors prescribed time away, a break from the ordinary that might give respite. Lawson remembers a trip to Nebraska, a summer week in Falmouth, trips designed in hopes her mother might recover an even keel and step back into her central role in the family. But it didn't seem to help. By 1964 Julia's forgetfulness had claimed the most essential tasks of daily life in her household, her domain. Baby diapers went unchanged, a child was left at school, meal times were skipped.

"Very little was known at the time about early Alzheimer's disease," Julie says. "They had a name for it, which was good, but it took them a long time to diagnose it, much longer than it would take today."

Julia was finally diagnosed with Alzheimer's disease in August of 1967. She was forty-three years old, and she would live another eleven years, much of it institutionalized in Foxborough State Hospital in Massachusetts. The gothic-looking compound, which closed in 1976 in a wave of deinstitutionalization, began life as the Massachusetts Hospital for Dipsomaniacs and Inebriates, and later became an inpatient psychiatric hospital.

"I can recall going in and seeing her in a bed, strapped, restrained, and medicated. They didn't know how to handle her at all." At the end, Julie says, she weighed eighty pounds, curled in the fetal position.

Looking back, Julie can see how the arc of the disease affected her family. In 2005 she shared that history with the Bipartisan Congressional Task Force on Alzheimer's Disease:

In 1967, with my mother's diagnosis of Alzheimer's disease, came the answer to much confusion in our lives. Julia and her identical twin, Agnes, were born in 1924 in Agawam, Massachusetts. Julia married her high school sweetheart and settled down to raise a family; little did she know that her future would be quite different. With the birth of my last sibling in 1964, my mom had noticeably progressed to forgetting her responsibilities as a mother, wife and homemaker. She forgot to change diapers, to make meals, to pick children up from school. She lost my dad's paycheck. Slowly, silently her love and ability to maintain a house disappeared.

Even though Mom was with us physically, her disappearing mind kept her from noticing what was going on for me or anyone else in the family. Confusion and fear were the prevailing emotions. Dad would get angry as he tried to rearrange the responsibilities of work and home. Uncertainty besieged his life as he questioned, "How could she forget her responsibilities like this?" These behaviors were so out of character for this young mother of ten who knew what it took to run a large household; she loved children and being a mom. This affected us all differently, but the common thread was the confusion that engulfed our lives.[4]

Something of a family historian, Julie pulls up a spreadsheet on her computer. There, she can track the march of Alzheimer's as it winds down the generations. The final entry for Julia Tatro Noonan is in April 1978, when she died from complications of end-stage Alzheimer's disease after many years of institutional care. There is another entry in the spreadsheet, however, that seems to foreshadow the era of genetic research into early onset Alzheimer's: Julia's identical twin, Agnes, began to show signs of the disease in 1975. Her battle would not last as long as Julia's, however; Agnes died in 1985 of lung cancer.

When Julie spoke before the congressional task force, she recounted a period of adaptation, of coming together as a family: "Now two young families were left without mothers; we were left to pick up the pieces and move forward, as each of us adapted to life after Alzheimer's disease had destroyed our family."[5] It seemed like the end of a long siege. But that was not to be the case, and the truth would be much more chilling: in 1992, at age forty-three, Julie's brilliant older sister, Fran Powers, began to show signs of forgetfulness. Her brother Butch and sister Maureen would follow.

Julie recalls that the familiar and haunting empty look in Fran's eyes reminded each sibling of the same vacant stare they received from their mother as children.[6] As Julie puts it now, she and her brothers and sisters recognized the savage truth: the disease that claimed their mother and aunt had reemerged in a new generation, which meant it was genetic. Fran was diagnosed with Alzheimer's disease in August of 1994, just a week before her forty-fifth birthday. Her children were fourteen and twelve.

Fran was well enough to speak about her condition before Congress on April 11, 1995, and Fran, her children, and Julie appeared on NBC's talk show *Leeza* in the fall of 1996.

Informed by her mother's illness, Fran took action while she could. "When she realized, 'I'm going down with this disease,' she went around and notified people" that she had early Alzheimer's, Julie says. Her friends and acquaintances in her community were grief stricken. "But Fran said, 'Hold on here. I'm not telling you this for your sympathy, I'm telling you because I need your help. I'm not going to remember things. If one of you could help me by calling me ten minutes before the appointment, or even a half-day before, it would help me enormously.'" As the disease took its relentless course, however, Fran continued to lose function, and by the winter of 2000, she was living in a nursing home in Pennsylvania.

In the PBS documentary *The Forgetting*, Fran makes a striking appearance. Handsome, with a shock of wavy white hair, she opens her blue eyes wide and gestures toward her sister and her husband. She caresses a face. At some points she laughs and seems delighted; at other points she seems withdrawn and absolutely terrified. Because of the family's pragmatic approach to the disease, and their wish to help educate others, allowing Fran to appear on camera was never an issue. Neither was the sort of candid approach that is evident in every bit of history that Julie recounts.

"I'm thankful—this time around with Butch—I'm thankful to be able to say, 'Look, he's going to have volatile behavior, let's just talk about it, let's be honest about it.' It blows people's minds that I want to talk about it and that I'm being this blunt," Julie says. "But I'm thankful for it on a continual basis when I look professionals in the eye and I can see that they're shocked that I am even talking about this."

Julie is, at her essence, a homegrown advocate for families and for Alzheimer's patients, recognizing that a disease that leaves no survivors beyond exhausted caregivers needs advocates who can demystify and educate. She has unpacked the story of the Noonan clan in public forums like the ABC program *20/20*, on PBS, and in Congress in order to save a few steps for someone else.

I think of the families like ourselves who have naively gone into facilities or a working relationship with a facility—because it is a working relationship, we're a team here and we have to care for this individual with Alzheimer's together. But the fact is that families go into these situations, and they have no idea that the patient is going to experience volatile behavior. They have watched the other losses and experienced them, and they may have even experienced volatile behavior in their own home with this patient, but they think it's about them. In the beginning stages of [early onset Alzheimer's], they're starting to check out, then they have clarity, then they check out again. There's nothing you can do to help them feel better. Medication can help. But I'm thankful that we have this knowledge and that we can share it with people.[7]

In *The Forgetting*, Fran can be seen standing in a specially made chair that allows her to move around her room but does not give her room to strike out at others. The nursing home had taken Fran's volatile behavior, and her needs, into account. Patients with early onset Alzheimer's can be volatile and angry, Julie explains, particularly in the early stages, when they have moments of clarity. In effect, she says, the disease causes a regression, and, like any preverbal toddler, the patient can get frustrated because he or she cannot communicate. "Fran had numerous instances where she was violent. She would be sent to one nursing home, and then another, and then another. She ended up with a record. It was cruel. Because, then, you know what happened? The nursing homes began to communicate and they would say, 'No, we can't take her.' Nobody wanted the responsibility. I don't blame them, because on the one hand, they have to protect their residents. But let's be honest about what kind of care they are giving in the first place."[8]

Although Fran died in December 2003 at 54, her life left Julie with important lessons, lessons that would come into play when her brother Butch's memory began to fail. The special chair, a type of walker, was a key part of her care, Julie says. "[Fran] was walking and very able to function," Julie says, but she was also volatile and would lash out at others. "So she was walking around and she had this bumper chair, and it extended out so she couldn't reach past it to get to somebody." The nursing home had met Fran exactly where she was in her disease progression: They adapted the care they provided to her needs.

Meeting Patients Where They Are

Julie returns to a central theme of patient care again and again: it's about meeting patients where they are. While this may sound like a simple concept, it is more complex in the setting of a nursing care facility that has to provide for a population with differing diagnoses and cope with training staff and maintaining proper standards while also meeting a budget.

Two years after Fran began showing signs of Alzheimer's in 1992, Maureen, the oldest sibling, went for tests. Her children had noticed an encroaching fog, a failure to remember, in the spring of 1994, when she was about to turn fifty-one. She received a definitive diagnosis of early onset Alzheimer's in 1995. This is when I met the family. It was a Friday, the day I usually had appointments at the Memory Disorders Clinic at Brigham and Women's Hospital. After seeing two patients earlier in the morning, the person at the desk told me my next appointment was waiting in one of the examining rooms. I opened the door and was totally surprised to see twelve people squeezed into the tiny room. Meet the Noonans! To this day the family reminds me of the jaw-dropping expression I had at the moment I saw this unexpected crowd instead of what I thought was my "next patient."

Because she was familiar with the trajectory of the disease, Maureen knew exactly how she wanted "to go out," as her sister Julie puts it. "Her children had a hard time finding placement for her, and when they did find placement, one of her wishes—and again, I'm sorry to say this and I know that I might offend some—she did not want to be fed if she could not feed herself. She was not asking anybody to kill her, but she was asking for an out. She said, 'If I can't take even my hand and reach it down and put it to my mouth, then please, don't you do it. That's my out.'"

Julie's eyes moisten as she recalls how her sister made the hardest decision of her life. "I wanted to honor this. We wanted to honor this." Julie understood she was working against a strong ethos embedded in the culture of medical care to keep a patient alive. "My mother lived for fifteen years, with relatively few bedsores for somebody who was bed-bound. But she was in the fetal position and she weighed probably eighty pounds. So we can keep our Alzheimer's patients alive—and I know some people do, and I'm not promoting that everyone is cut from the same mold—but my sister Maureen watched my mom and knew what she wanted and asked for it."

Although Maureen had not put her end-of-life request in writing, her children wanted to honor her wishes and searched for a new care facility that would agree. "So they had to find a new place," Julie says, "and a hospice nurse was opening a home for hospice patients, and they allowed Maureen to move in. She was bedbound at this point, but she had a wonderful room with a bathroom off of it, kind of tucked in the corner of the house. It had its own entrance, so her kids could come and go and her grandchildren would play on the floor of the living room. They had music going and they could gather around her there. I'm sure it was just the way Maureen would have wanted to go." She died on November 23, 2001.

Alzheimer's is hard on caregivers as well, because spouses and children coordinating round-the-clock care let their own medical appointments lapse and pay less attention to the wear and tear on their own bodies. Tragically, this held true for Maureen's husband, Dick. He died suddenly in December of 1999, five years after Maureen's diagnosis. The official cause was a heart attack, but many in the Noonan family attribute this additional loss to Alzheimer's.

When Julie Noonan spoke before Congress in 2005, she was candid about the wreckage:

> I speak to you today with firsthand knowledge of the fear of losing my mind and of wondering at every turn if the actions I exhibit speak of a future with Alzheimer's disease. I live daily with knowing that this disease not only removes the many memories of a person's mind, but like a tornado, destroys all relationships in its path and changes the directions of those relationships forever. Therefore, having lived almost my entire life gaining firsthand knowledge of the destruction of Alzheimer's disease, the thought of putting my own children through this was more than I could bear. Once the fear of getting the disease outweighed my ability to redirect my thoughts and the suspension of my life outweighed the enjoyment of living my life, I knew it was time to find out if I was a carrier of the mutation.

Genetic Testing: A Highly Personal Choice

By 2003, Julie felt herself straining to remember the tasks of daily life. She was balancing her own family obligations and negotiating a landscape of caretaking and grief. Maureen had died, and Fran was near death. Julie wondered: Did she carry the genetic mutation for early onset Alzheimer's? Was she next? With the availability of predictive genetic testing for the mutation that causes Alzheimer's disease in this family I organized a family gathering at Brigham and Women's Hospital to discuss the myriad of knotty issues associated with genetic testing. It was a weekend, and we booked a large conference room on the ground floor. Branches of the family flew in from all over the country in what was a large meeting of the clans. Blood was drawn and swabs were taken. I spoke to the group and emphasized that getting tested for the mutation is a highly personal choice, that no one should coerce another person to get tested, that the results are highly private even in this hypercommunicative family, and each of them needed to be fully aware of the unintended consequences of genetic testing. Julie was very aware of one of the most important consequences: the effect of the genetic news on one's children and siblings. The knowledge that something deadly lies in one's genes is like nothing else—it reveals not only one's own fate, but also, if the gene was passed to a child, the fate of the child. In Julie's case, her twenty-year-old daughter wanted no part of this family burden she had never asked for, and did not want her mother to be tested. That feeling is common among younger adults, who often fail to see—or don't want to see—the finitude of life.

What changed Julie's mind about testing was what Julie observed when her brother John got his test results. John was certain he wanted to be tested and bravely walked in for his results with Julie by his side. When he was told he did not have the Alzheimer gene, John's expression and demeanor changed in way that Julie had not seen in years. As if released from chains, he was transformed; he suddenly seemed lighter than air. Julie said, "I want that feeling." In June 2003 she asked for her test results and was told she was negative. She did not carry the genetic flaw that had claimed so much of her family.

"I thank God I am not a carrier," Julie told Congress in her 2005 testimony, "but sadly enough I have lost four family members to this disease. Besides Mom and her twin sister, my sisters Maureen and Frances have lost the battle, and we are in the process of losing my dear brother Malcolm. In addition, we do not know who of the next generation is living with this time bomb. This genetic legacy has had a different effect on each of us with the weight and responsibility. . . . [W]e have decided to band together to fight this disease."

If the family history seems particularly vivid on this fall day in her kitchen, it is because her brother Malcolm, known as Butch, is entering a new phase in his battle with the disease. The third child of Julia Tatro Noonan to enter the long twilight of decline associated with the disease, Butch had participated in a family study at the National Institutes of Health and had watched his sisters' decline. So it came as no surprise, Julie says, that he recognized the changes in his own personality as early as 1995. "He is amazing. He is twenty years AA [Alcoholics Anonymous], so he is not just a recovering alcoholic but a practicing recovering alcoholic. He applied the program to his life and did emotional work. He would see himself. He would see his deficits. He was in school to become a licensed mental health therapist. So of course he didn't know he had it, but he just felt like his brain wasn't working like it should work. That's what he would say. And so he could see it coming, but he had a peace about it."

Butch had worked as a chef and a plumber, and then had returned to school and become a licensed mental health therapist. Although the symptoms of the disease had begun to emerge, he was able to work as a counselor. "He did get to finish his education," Julie says. "He was actually employed for a while as a mental health counselor. And he was damn good at it. He got to succeed."

He had to resign from his job in 2003 as the disease took its toll, and Julie and Butch's wife, Sheila, are touring full-time care facilities as his decline accelerates. He has moments of recognition and moments when elements of his personality and his past bubble to the surface. Julie describes a car trip with Butch to the neurologist, when music made a connection and she had an insight into a way to reach her brother. "We were all listening to a sixties program on satellite radio, and there's Butch, bopping to the music. He was singing away and I said, 'OK. So this is the music we need for Butch, not whatever my mother used to sing when we were kids.' He was totally grooving on it."

The Search for a Nursing Home

The decision to put Butch in a nursing home was hard, Julie says, but she is determined to see that Sheila will get the support she needs. She does not want to see another Noonan spouse claimed by the burden of caretaking. What signs pointed the family toward nursing home care? At fifty-seven, Butch is still strong. Episodes of volatile behavior are typically harder to control in younger patients with early onset Alzheimer's. And, in a course that is typical of the disease, Butch does not know what his physical needs are. He is disconnected from the physical signals his bladder sends to his brain when he needs to urinate, so he is peeing in the wrong places. "Some of that could be cleared up with twenty-four-hour care," Julie explains, "with professionals who change shifts, who get a break, who aren't emotionally attached."

So the search for a suitable nursing home has begun, and Julie is sobered by what she has found—and solemn about her glimpse into the future of any frail elder who will need around-the-clock care, whether for Alzheimer's disease or another ailment. The quality of facilities is mixed, she notes, and the economic equation is daunting.

Her goal is to find a nursing home that will meet Butch where he is in the course of the disease, respect the family's visitation schedule, and honor any end-of-life instructions. And, of course, she wants a basic level of cleanliness and a reasonable staff level, with aides and administrators and others who are not burned out—who see the humanity of the population they're working with. But, as her notes attest, that model of care is not always easy to find.

In an entry dated Oct. 16, 2008, she wrote the following notes about her impressions:

> [Nursing home name deleted] is presently caring for three residents under the age of sixty and their oldest resident is one hundred and two! Right now fourteen percent of the population is male. There are sixty-five of what they call "apartments," which are basically individual rooms about three hundred and fifty square feet and five hundred twenty-five square feet, and residents can have their own furniture. Rooms are grouped in quads. There is twenty-four-hour visiting. The front door is locked from eight p.m. to eight a.m., but you ring into the quad your family member lives in and they will let you in. Upon moving to [name deleted] the first thirty days they are assigned a Transitional Companion: this person's responsibility is to help the new resident adjust to the new environment. This would be the same three people for round-the-clock care. They would assess day by day as to how the new resident is adjusting. Volatile behavior will generate an evaluation from their staff and include family input. They will look at areas like medication, illness, and environment to see what is causing the problem behavior. A psych evaluation is the last option. [Name deleted] would honor any living will Butch has established, including not being fed if he can't feed himself. Because [name deleted] is an assisted living facility, if Butch was to stay . . . until the very end, the Visiting Nurses Association or hospice would have to be hired as an outside source. We need to find out how this service would get paid for. Would Medicare pay for this?

Her entries continued. For Oct. 21, 2008, she wrote:

> Well, we looked at two more nursing homes today. [Name deleted] is located next to a schoolyard, and listening to the children play was a sweet sound when we entered the facility. The lady's room public bathroom was dirty. [Name deleted] was willing to try but when we asked how they would handle volatile behavior they said the staff is trained to handle this behavior and that the first two weeks are usually difficult transition for new residents. They also said they have a responsibility to keep all residents safe as well as the person with the volatile behavior, and if the behavior continued they will Section Twelve him (send him to a psych ward). I asked them how they would know if they

could handle him and they said they would have a team come to his house to evaluate his level using the Global Deterioration Scale, one being normal and ten being total care. But they strongly recommended that we place him in a psych hospital for evaluation before being placed anywhere. This screams to me big time "We really can't handle him!" Upon exiting the elevator and before entering into the Alzheimer's unit it smelt like . . . crap. The unit itself smelt like urine. As we were walking through the unit the staff basically ignored us, no one said "Hi" or made eye contact with us. And one of the janitors was emptying the trash and making very loud banging noises and when one of the residents asked him to quiet down he just smiled at them like they were stupid.

Her narrative continued with another entry for Oct. 21, 2008:

[Name deleted] has wonderful murals inside and out. This facility was overall cleaner and the Alzheimer's disease unit didn't smell like urine or crap. The hallways were carpeted and the unit seemed cheerier. Once again the staff basically ignored us, no one said "Hi" or made eye contact with us as we walked through the unit. When we sat down after the tour I asked the MSW how they would handle volatile behavior and she said (without hesitation), "Not well."

Julie shares her impressions candidly because it is part of the family ethos. The Noonan clan has rallied and organized to raise money for research and to further the public's understanding of early onset Alzheimer's disease. (She jokes that their crack organizational skills come from family trips to the beach long ago—"You get the towels, you pack the lunches—for ten kids!") They have testified before Congress, appeared on television, and allowed scientists to bank their DNA and brain tissue in the interest of research.

As Julie told Congress that spring day in 1995, "As a family we believe in the extreme need for research." While she is excited about scientific advances, she pushes for awareness of the impact of seventy-seven million baby boomers—who are cresting into retirement and old age—on the nation's healthcare system. Knowing well that nursing home care costs about $50,000 a year—and hospice and visiting nurse care costs extra—she pressed Congress for an increase in funds for research. "From my vantage point, finding a cure, which is closer than it ever has been before, is a more sensible option than to pay for long-term care for seventy-seven million baby boomers."

There is perhaps no greater tribute to the organizational skills and inspiring style of the Noonans than the annual fund-raising bicycle ride called the Memory Ride, which they founded in 1997. The event is approaching $2 million in total funds raised. The cyclists travel a rugged route over two, and sometimes three, days through the green New England countryside to their destination in Boston. Seeing the lead bikers coming up Beacon Street on the final stretch toward the Massachusetts State House is truly a tears-of-joy moment.

Several years after the Memory Ride began, I began to meet the cyclists at their campgrounds in western Massachusetts, where they rested for the night and prepared for the second arduous day's trek back to Boston. This particular year, a simple dinner was set up in the Fitchburg High School cafeteria. After saying a few words of thanks to the group, I walked outside to see a hillside dotted with tents. Only a little light was left in the sky. I looked down the dark road along which the bikers would begin their trek the next morning. A few streetlights trailed off in the distance, and then the road went dark. It made me think of the road the Alzheimer patient travels. For us, at nightfall the ride stops, and we rejuvenate ourselves in the soft, incandescent glow of lanterns and the circle of tent light and the comfort of friends. But for the Alzheimer patient, the road just keeps going, on into the darkness.

ALZHEIMER'S DISEASE ON THE WORLD STAGE

The Reagan Family's Experience

Five years after he left the White House after two terms as president, Ronald Reagan wrote a letter to the American people that was heartfelt, if stark, in its simplicity. It marked the end of his public life.

Nov. 5, 1994

My fellow Americans, I have recently been told that I am one of the millions of Americans who will be afflicted with Alzheimer's disease.

Upon learning this news, Nancy and I had to decide whether as private citizens we would keep this a private matter or whether we would make this news known in a public way. In the past, Nancy suffered from breast cancer and I had my cancer surgeries. We found through our open disclosures we were able to raise public awareness. We were happy that as a result, many more people underwent testing. They were treated in early stages and able to return to normal, healthy lives.

So now we feel it is important to share it with you. In opening our hearts, we hope this might promote greater awareness of this condition. Perhaps it will encourage a clearer understanding of the individuals and families who are affected by it.

At the moment I feel just fine. I intend to live the remainder of the years God gives me on this Earth doing the things I have always done. I will continue to share life's journey with my beloved Nancy and my family. I plan to enjoy the great outdoors and stay in touch with my friends and supporters.

Unfortunately, as Alzheimer's disease progresses, the family often bears a heavy burden. I only wish there was some way I could spare Nancy from this painful experience. When the time comes, I am confident that with your help she will face it with faith and courage.

In closing, let me thank you, the American people, for giving me the great honor of allowing me to serve as your president. When the Lord calls me home, whenever that day may be, I will leave with the greatest love for this country of ours and eternal optimism for its future.

I now begin the journey that will lead me into the sunset of my life. I know that for America there will always be a bright dawn ahead.

Thank you, my friends. May God always bless you.[9]

The record does not reflect who wrote this letter—whether it was a gifted speechwriter like Peggy Noonan (not part of the Noonan family with Alzheimer's disease), or Nancy Reagan, or the former president himself. But the letter—the public acknowledgement that a beloved leader faced a long decline—was a watershed moment in the history of Alzheimer's. Certainly, celebrities had been diagnosed before: Actress Rita Hayworth died of Alzheimer's in 1987 at age sixty-eight, and her daughter, Yasmin Khan, became a regular figure on the fund-raising circuit, hosting galas and speaking at conferences. But Reagan, somehow, seemed different.

"Reagan was the ultimate 'regular guy' even though he was a masterful leader and user of power," says Dr. Leslie Feldman, professor of political science at Hofstra University in New York. "The disclosure of his Alzheimer's made him even more so—and I think part of the reason they went public was so they could raise money for Alzheimer's research. Also, they wanted the world to know why he was dropping out of sight. This way *they* could control it. He was an actor (and Nancy an actress) and it was time to exit the stage—and they knew when to get off. They wanted to get off how and when they wanted, so that people would remember Reagan's image as the cowboy and statesman. The greatest world leaders—Mikhail Gorbachev and Margaret Thatcher—had respect for him, but it was his image as the regular guy, even in his B movies, that people seemed to relate to."[10]

Public reaction was sadness and compassion, along with a renewed discussion of a disease that had once seemed obscure. By acknowledging the disease, the Reagans helped bring it out of the shadows of shame and grief. (Unlike cancer and other chronic illnesses, Alzheimer's leaves no survivors to mount races for a cure—and caretakers are often too exhausted.) Fundraising for Alzheimer's increased, according to press reports, from $146 million in 1990 to $650 million in 2006.

Reagan's popularity was evident: He had drubbed his opponents in two elections—the second won by a landslide—and brought with him a sense of sweeping change and, for many, the freshening winds of a conservative revolution. He also gave voice to a feeling of possibility, and his speeches were masterful in painting long-held American ideals in broad strokes. In his Farewell Address to the Nation from the Oval Office on January 11, 1989, he summoned up a 359-year-old image woven into the fabric of colonial America: the "shining city on a hill." The phrase came from a sermon given by John Winthrop to Puritans aboard the ship *Arbella*, who would soon land and settle the Massachusetts Bay Colony. It was his last speech as president. About to turn seventy-eight, Reagan seemed in good form:

> I've spoken of the shining city all my political life, but I don't know if I ever quite communicated what I saw when I said it. But in my mind it was a tall, proud city built on rocks stronger than oceans, windswept, God-blessed, and teeming with people of all kinds living in harmony and peace, a city with free ports that hummed with commerce and creativity, and if there had to be city walls, the walls had doors and the doors were open to anyone with the will and the heart to get here. That's how I saw it and see it still.
>
> And how stands the city on this winter night? More prosperous, more secure, and happier than it was eight years ago. But more than that; after 200 years, two centuriees, she still stands strong and true on the granite ridge, and her glow has held steady no matter what storm. And she's still a beacon, still a magnet for all who must have freedom, for all the pilgrims from all the lost places who are hurtling through the darkness, toward home.[11]

Knowing what we know now about Reagan's final journey, it is a poignant image to come back to: hurtling through the darkness, toward home.

Reagan highlighted small moments and invested them with big meaning. He did not see himself as the Great Communicator, a nickname bestowed on him because of his breezy, avuncular style of speaking that seemed to connect in an elemental way with his audience. Instead, as he said in his farewell address, he saw himself as something of a conduit for ideas and stories that stood for something grander.

After the letter revealing the Alzheimer's diagnosis was released, the family kept a tight lock on the former president's privacy. In the winter of 2003, his son Ron opened up, however briefly, with a public television interviewer. "Well, the terrible thing about Alzheimer's is, of course, is it robs the victim of the memories, the tapestry of memories and recollections that constitute the self in so many ways, and not only does the victim lose their own sense of self and their sense of place within their sort of social continuum and the family but the people around them, the loved ones, begin to question whether this is the same person we always knew."

A month before Reagan's death in June 2004, Nancy Reagan talked to Terence Smith, a correspondent with the *NewsHour with Jim Lehrer*. In the interview, the former first lady leveled with the public about the grief Alzheimer's leaves in its wake. "Ronnie's long journey has finally taken him to a distant place where I can no longer reach him," she said. "I think that's probably the hardest part. Those with Alzheimer's are on a rocky path that only goes downhill. Because of this, I'm determined to do what I can to save other families from this pain."[12]

She advocated broader use of stem cell research to treat Alzheimer's and other diseases, a position she held even though it marked a departure from Bush administration policy and from the conservative orthodoxy of the day.

David Shenk, in his book *The Forgetting*, raises the question of whether Reagan had Alzheimer's while in office. "Yes and no," he writes. "Without a doubt, he was on his way to getting the disease, which develops over many years. But it is equally clear that there was not yet nearly enough decline in function to support even a tentative diagnosis. Reagan's mind was well within the realm of normal functioning."[13]

The attempt on Reagan's life by John Hinckley Jr. on March 30, 1981, clearly took a lot out of him—more than the public knew at the time. His diary entry for that day reads, in part: "Getting shot hurts. Still my fear was growing because no matter how hard I tried to breathe it seemed I was getting less & less air. I focused on that tiled ceiling [in the emergency room at George Washington University Hospital] and prayed."[14] He was discharged from the hospital on Saturday, April 12. Gingerly, he began to resume his work schedule as he recuperated in the White House. The abridged volume of his diaries, edited by historian Douglas Brinkley and released in 2007, contains no suggestion of cognitive impairment after the shooting—or at the end of his term in January 1989, when he was about to turn seventy-eight. He was tired, of course, as he recovered from his wounds and began to take up the demands of a head of state.

Monday, April 13

I'm beginning to have a work schedule. We meet in the mornings in the treaty room. It feels good to be whittling at the problems. Afternoon is still nap time and bed time follows dinner by about ½ an hour.

Saturday, April 18

A nice quiet day—no emergencies, slept in late but still managed an afternoon nap. Wrote a draft of a letter to Brezhnev. Don't know whether I'll send it but enjoyed putting some thoughts down on paper. 9 P.M. and we're off to bed.[15]

Yet by April 23, 1981, Reagan was meeting with Senator Howard Baker "re the AWAC's sale to Saudi Arabia & the fuss being kicked up about it,"[16] and appended to that day's diary entry is a letter that Reagan wrote to Leonid Brezhnev by hand, in which he makes an appeal for the release of Natan Sharansky, who was being held in a Soviet prison.

And by Monday, May 4, 1981, Reagan seemed back in the swing of things, enjoying "a beautiful spring day" by taking lunch in the White House solarium and then sun-bathing for "about an hour."[17]

After a dinner for the Reagans given by Edmund Morris, the historian who was chosen to be Reagan's official biographer, Morris asked guests to write down their impressions of Ronald Reagan. (The dinner, on November 15, 1987, was held in Morris's townhouse, and included a number of writers in formal dress.) Morris later recorded their impressions in his biography, *Dutch: A Memoir of Ronald Reagan*:

[Robert K. Massie] Somehow, he was both there—very much there—and not there at the same time. I was surprised by his affability and vigor. He is an extremely nice fellow and the reports I've read or heard about his "senility" are absurd. . . . What bothered me about Reagan was his lack of curiosity as to what we did and what we thought about the world. There was a kind of impenetrable curtain hanging between us and the President. . . . But I must say—and perhaps it is the invisible crown all Presidents wear—that he seemed to dwarf all of the twelve men currently scrambling round the country, trying to take his place.[18]

As his second term came to an end in mid-November 1988, Reagan required detailed briefing cards prepared for him by his White House staff—all for a ten-minute private conversation with his longtime ally Prime Minister Margaret Thatcher of Britain. Journalist Nicholas Wapshott, who memorialized the Reagan-Thatcher friendship and alliance in his book *Ronald Reagan and Margaret Thatcher: A Political Marriage*, writes that Reagan took the set of cards, titled "Points to be made at one-on-one with Prime Minister Margaret Thatcher," to a meeting that included Thatcher, a note taker, and British foreign affairs adviser Charles Powell.

"The president had become so reliant on scripted prompts to get him through meetings that his staff left nothing to chance, even down to the opening remark: 'I am delighted to see you back in Washington,'" writes Wapshott, who unearthed the cards at the Reagan presidential library. "His next talking point was, 'There is so much talk about change in the Soviet Union and what it means for the West. We, together, have been the driving force for change over the last eight years.'"[19]

The prompts on the cards ended with the most basic final question imaginable: "I know you have a full agenda to cover with me. Is there anything you would like to raise now before we ask the others to join us?" One imagines the aging president and former actor losing his grip on facts and unable to follow the give-and-take of a diplomatic conversation with another head of state, but still being able to call on a skill that had long served him well: hitting his mark, reading his dialogue.

Morris noticed changes in Reagan when the former president, then eighty-one, returned to the White House to accept the Presidential Medal of Freedom on January 13, 1993, in the waning days of the Bush administration—and eight days before Bill Clinton was inaugurated.

Morris listened to Reagan's short acceptance speech and noted that his voice was rough and his delivery was slow. Then, in the receiving line, Morris was dismayed by Reagan's behavior: "Afterward, in the receiving line, he took my hand and nodded with patent lack of recognition. His eyes were dulled by the confusion that had been lowering upon him since our trip to Tampico, eight months before. Or so I thought. . . . Well, it had to happen, I told myself as I moved on to the champagne table. Dutch finally stopped recognizing me."

But the next day, a Reagan aide called Morris and said that on the flight back to Los Angeles, Reagan had remarked, "I saw Edmund in the reception line this morning. And you know what? I think he's waiting for me to die before he publishes his book."

Although Reagan had been sharp enough to make a joke in early

1993, less than a month later he gave "his first public evidence of cognitive frailty," Morris writes. "I attended his eighty-second birthday celebration at the Ronald Reagan Presidential Library in Simi Valley, along with several hundred other guests, including Margaret Thatcher, and we all froze when he toasted her twice, at length, and in exactly the same words. There was nothing we could do but give her two standing ovations, and not look too closely at Nancy Reagan's stricken face, while Dutch stood obliviously smiling."[20]

Morris, a respected historian known for his biographies of President Theodore Roosevelt, was criticized for his unconventional approach in *Dutch*. Yet his observations, based on close study of Reagan for a number of years, cannot be easily dismissed. "Remember, Morris was the official Reagan biographer who was so confused by the complex yet simple Reagan that he put himself into the biography as a fictional character," says Feldman, the Hofstra presidential scholar. "While he was criticized for this, I still think the book can provide excellent insights into Reagan."[21]

Margaret Thatcher and the Last Taboo

Margaret Thatcher often shared the world stage with Ronald Reagan during the 1980s. Known as the Iron Lady, her conservative ideology reshaped the economic policies of the United Kingdom, much as Reagan had ushered in an era of tax cuts and "supply side" economics in the United States. Elected the first woman leader of the Conservative Party in February 1975, she had a long run as prime minister from 1979 to 1990.[22]

Reagan and Thatcher both charted their rise to political power as the Vietnam War drew to a close in the 1970s, and forged a conservative path in reaction to the social and geopolitical tumult all around.

She would share another experience with Reagan: a battle with dementia that would be waged, in part, in the public eye.

The two rising political figures hit it off when they first met in April 1975. Thatcher had just been elected head of the Conservative Party and Reagan was a former governor of California eager to show that he had foreign policy experience as he flirted with the idea of a presidential run. Reagan was in England to meet with figures in the Labour and Conservative parties, and while Labour officials were somewhat bemused by the ex-governor, the session with Thatcher had the tang of history.

When Reagan was inaugurated in January 1981, Thatcher sent a letter expressing hope for a working partnership.

1981 Jan 20 Tu

Dear Mr. President,

May I send you my congratulations, and those of my colleagues in the British Government, on your inauguration as President of the United States. You face a formidable task of leadership at a dangerous time. But your inauguration is a symbol of hope for the Alliance, and you can depend on our confidence and support as we work together to meet the challenges of the 1980s.

I look forward to renewing our friendship when we meet in Washington next month, and to consolidating the close relationship between our two countries.

With best wishes
Warm personal regards,
Yours sincerely,
Margaret Thatcher

"Several sources record that President-elect Reagan was touched by the warmth of this message," the Thatcher Foundation noted in an editorial comment appended to this letter.[23]

In a confidential cable to Thatcher, declassified in 1997, Reagan wrote to Thatcher about her impending visit to the United States in February 1981 and sounded notes of friendship and collaboration.

You are indeed right that we share a very special concern for democracy and for liberty. That is the essence of the special relationship between our two countries, and it is similarly an excellent basis for inaugurating an extended period of co-operation and close consultation between your government and my administration.

It is with greatest anticipation that I look forward to your arrival here and to the opportunity for extensive discussions on the broad range of world issues with which we must deal in partnership.

Ronald Reagan[24]

That visit, from February 25 to March 1, cemented the friendship. Sir Nicholas Henderson, the British ambassador to the United States, recorded their mutual admiration in his diary. "Before the visit they had both decided, as I know from what they each said to me, that they liked each other: this was on the basis of their two earlier meetings, a few years back, and of their similar political and economic policies (government off the backs of the people; greater incentives to industry; everything for the individual) and of the warm message Mrs. T had sent immediately [*sic*] the election results were known," Henderson writes. "[James] Brady, the White House Press Secretary, said after the visit was over that it had been 'difficult to prise them apart.' This was fortunate."[25]

Thatcher was known as the Iron Lady for her tough stance against the Soviet Union, and it was a label she wore proudly as she forged an alliance with Reagan on defense during the waning days of the Cold War.

"I don't think Thatcher was beloved in Britain the way Reagan was in the United States," says Stanislao Pugliese, professor of European studies at Hofstra University. "She did win three successive elections and she did transform the political landscape, but I don't think that she had the same kind of personality and relationship with the people of Britain that Reagan had with the American people." Pugliese, who was part of a Hofstra conference on Thatcher, does see some similarities between the Iron Lady and the Great Communicator, however, and believes that they drew ideological strength from one another. "They both saw themselves as political outsiders. Both came from the right wing of their parties, Reagan as a governor and former actor, and Lady Thatcher as the daughter of a grocer, a member of the lower middle class. They both always had this kind of latent, subterranean resentment toward the elite and toward the political class."[26] After she resigned as prime minister in November 1990, she remained a force in politics, giving lectures and writing three books—*The Downing Street Years* (1993), *The Path to Power* (1995) and *Statecraft* (2002). After a series of small strokes in 2002, she withdrew from the public stage.

But, as her daughter, Carol, would later write, her family had begun worrying about the state of her health and memory two years earlier. In an article in the *Mail on Sunday*, Carol Thatcher recalls where she was when she realized her mother's memory had begun to falter.[27] The two were having lunch, at Carol's invitation, at the Mandarin Oriental Hotel in Knightsbridge, overlooking Hyde Park. As Carol writes, "It was such a rare mother-and-daughter occasion, I relished it. Mum was hardly a 'lady who lunched' and I'd had to wait months to find a space in her diary when we could get together. It's not always easy to make polite, lunchtime conversation with a mother who for decades has had international leaders and statesmen to engage with in potential world-changing discussions."

Their discussion turned to Bosnia, and Carol expected her formidable mother to begin a "characteristic monologue." Instead, the former prime minister became confused, muddled her history of the

Bosnian war with that of the Falklands—history that she had very much been a part of. "I almost fell off my chair," Carol writes. "Watching her struggle with her words and her memory, I couldn't believe it. She was in her 75th year but I had always thought of her as ageless, timeless and 100 percent cast-iron damage-proof."[28] Like many children noticing short-term memory loss in a parent for the first time, the episode was a benchmark. Carol would come back to that lunch, and to the clinical significance of what she saw in her mother, again and again as she watched her mother's notable mind fade. "The contrast was all the more striking because, until that point, she'd always had a memory like a website."[29]

That memory was a source of pride for her mother, who was always able to draw on her command of history, economics, and facts in the fabled debates that occurred in Parliament during the Prime Minister's Questions. Cradle of oratory that they are, these sessions are no place for the tongue-tied, and Thatcher could soar.

"During Prime Minister's Questions, she could rise from the front bench in an economic debate and recite the rate of inflation all the way back to William Gladstone without a note," Carol writes. "From the fateful day of our lunch, telltale signs that something wasn't quite right began to emerge."[30]

Thatcher began to have difficulty remembering appointments, and repeatedly asked the same questions. As her daughter documents, the earliest manifestations of dementia can be difficult to cope with because family members are still adjusting to the very fact of the disease. "That's the worst thing about dementia: it gets you every time. Sufferers look and act the same but beneath the familiar exterior something quite different is going on. They're in another world and you cannot enter."[31]

There were moments of clarity, when her long-term memory filled in gaps and Thatcher recalled the rationing during World War II or conversations with Mikhail Gorbachev. "It was a case of classic dementia, coupled with a series of mini-strokes," Carol writes. "What was most galling was that there was nothing I could do: this cruel disease takes its own course."[32]

After her husband, Denis, died in 2003, Thatcher had to be reminded over and over again that he was gone. "Losing Dad, however, was truly awful for Mum, not least because her dementia meant she kept forgetting he was dead. I had to keep giving her the bad news over and over again. Every time it finally sank in that she had lost her husband of more than 50 years, she'd look at me sadly and say, 'Oh,' as I struggled to compose myself. 'Were we all there?' she'd ask softly. These days, my mother cannot remember every detail of her time at No. 10 or particular pieces of legislation she created but she has told me she thinks her place in history is assured."[33]

The reaction in Britain to Carol Thatcher's disclosures was scathing. Amanda Platell, former press secretary for Conservative leader William Hague, was unforgiving in a column written for the *Mail* in August 2008. "The Iron Lady perhaps did not always make the most natural and attentive of mothers. But however difficult it must have been at times for Carol to live in her mother's shadow, I couldn't help but feel saddened yesterday to discover that she has written an opportunistic book in which she describes the terrible dementia Lady Thatcher is now suffering. To me and to many who admired or loved her mother, it felt not only like a terrible invasion of an old woman's privacy, but a personal betrayal. There's a time and a place for such memoirs. But this was not it. Too soon, Carol. Too much detail."[34]

For years, Platell writes, those close to Thatcher kept her condition a secret. Platell acknowledged that she had noticed that Thatcher was losing "her steel trap of a mind" years before, while Denis Thatcher was still alive. It was during a speech to fellow Conservative Party members, Platell writes, when she began to lose her train of thought. "Almost imperceptibly, Denis, sitting next to her, tapped the table several times and said softly under his breath, 'repeating, repeating.' It was his signal to her to stop. And she did. No one in the audience that night breathed a word about what they had witnessed. Which makes it all the more perplexing that a daughter should think it acceptable not only to reveal her mother's most intimate secrets to the world, but also to make money out of it."[35]

Pugliese reflects on Thatcher's legacy: "I don't think, looking back on it now with the perspective of more than ten years, that her impact on British society was as great as we thought when she first left office. But it could be that the perspective on her has mellowed over time. Maybe the ordinary people in the street have more sympathy for her because of her medical condition, but I think it is a very different kind of image today than when she left office."[36]

Jane Gross, a longtime reporter for the *New York Times* who now writes "The New Old Age" blog for nytimes.com, raised the conflicting issues at the heart of the debate in Britain: "On the one hand, it does seem to violate a proud woman's privacy to describe the sad diminishment of her formidable powers, particularly when she doesn't seem capable—as President Reagan was—of making the disclosures herself. On the other hand, it makes her poignantly human. Many of our parents will, in the end, suffer what she is suffering; many of us will, too, when our turn comes. So why the secrecy and shame?"[37]

Many Britons expressed sympathy in posts on the Web site Mail-Online, arguing in favor of finally speaking openly about dementia and Alzheimer's, long-held taboos. Gross summed it up neatly when she wrote, "As a friend of mine put it, 'If you refuse to talk about it, you're treating it as something shameful,' once the common response to cancer."

The reactions of Reagan and Thatcher to their encroaching dementia illustrate extremes: honest disclosure on the one hand, and shame and secrecy on the other. But when public figures come forward to talk about their condition, it can spur everything from fresh dialogue in the public square about their illness to a renewed commitment to research. In Reagan's case, his wife, Nancy, became an exception to the Republican Party stance on embryonic stem cell research, declaring her support. Thatcher, who was a patron of the Alzheimer's Research Trust, could have advanced understanding of dementia. (While Thatcher has not been officially diagnosed with Alzheimer's—or at least no such diagnosis has been publicly disclosed—her symptoms mirror the decline typical for an Alzheimer's patient.)

As Alexander Chancellor, a columnist for the *Guardian* newspaper in the UK, observed, it meant a lot when British author Terry Pratchett told the world that he had early onset Alzheimer's and described what it felt like on radio and television in September 2008. "Like Reagan," Chancellor writes, "he disclosed his condition at an early enough stage to be able to talk lucidly and with good humour about it. This is a spirit that gives encouragement to the afflicted and comfort to the carers, while also stimulating public interest and support."[38]

Patricia Garamendi: Tragedy, Love, and Hope

The story of Patricia Garamendi and her mother pulses with life, hope, and newfound connections. Trained as a lawyer, married to Lieutenant Governor John Garamendi of California, Patricia has taken her ninety-year-old mother, who has Alzheimer's disease, into her own home on the agriculture-rich delta of the Sacramento River to give her a gentle and dignified sunset.

In fact, Patricia has put her considerable public policy experience—and her innate resilience—to work in drawing attention to the ravages of the disease and the need for more research, more funding, and early screening. She has a varied background in public service, starting with a stint as a Peace Corps volunteer (along with her husband) in Ethiopia.

During the Clinton administration, she was associate director of the Peace Corps, overseeing twenty-one thousand volunteers in ninety-one countries. She has also served as deputy administrator for the Foreign Agriculture Service of the US Department of Agriculture. Now she balances her roles as mother of six children and caretaker for the family matriarch, Merle Wilkinson, with her job as agriculture specialist for the California Exposition and State Fair.

Patricia's life is busy, to say the least. But she has never regretted her decision to care for her mother independently, outside of an institutional setting—and remains undaunted even in the face of a fresh tragedy that upended the family's life in January of 2008. Her mother had been living in her own home, surrounded by family photos and memories, supported by caregivers who helped her adapt to daily life. With an eye to dignity, Patricia worked with those caring for her mother to paint a full picture, to help them get to know everything from the proper drug regimen to the names of children, grandchildren, and great-grandchildren.

And in 2007, when Patricia Garamendi wrote an essay for *care ADvantage*, a publication of the Alzheimer's Foundation of America, things seemed to be going well. In the essay, she described the picturesque scene and the cascade of bittersweet emotions as she arrived at her mother's home:

> The sun reflected off the stained glass window as I quietly pushed open that old familiar door. I walked slowly through the living room and down the hall and was overcome by memories of a grand lady who always had the front door decorated with the seasons. Through the years, whatever the holiday, she would be in the kitchen, cooking our favorite dishes as she awaited our arrival with great anticipation. Around her home are memories of our family life, childhood photos of her three daughters, the cracked teacup that had belonged to her mother, my paintings that she proudly displayed, pictures with all of her grandchildren hugging her. I wondered, how would things be today? As I rounded the corner, there she was, cuddled in her afghan looking out the window. "Mama, it's me, your daughter Patti," I said. Slowly, she turned and, as she focused on my face, her eyes began to fill with tears. Her face lighted up as our souls touched and her hand touched her throat, a sign that she was filled with emotion.[39]

Merle was comfortably ensconced in her own home, and her daughters, caregivers, and extended family were intent on maintaining every vestige of connection, every possible link to her interior world that might elicit a spark of recognition. "We had been fortunate as a family to be able to keep Mama in her own home, surrounded by family pictures and memories of a lifetime of happy events," Patricia recalled later in a speech for the Alzheimer's Foundation of America Concepts in Care Conference. "We appreciated how important it was to help her caregivers to understand the special needs of those with Alzheimer's disease, and how important it was to maintain her dignity in helping her dress, and fix her hair, and apply her make-up so that she was ready to start her day by looking like herself and maintaining the pride she always took in her appearance."[40]

But on January 6, 2008, the unthinkable happened: a fire roared through Merle's home in the night, leaving chaos, death, and destruction. A relative was overcome by smoke and died trying to rescue Merle from the burning house. Another caregiver escaped but was hospitalized with severe burns to her ankles and left hand—burns that would later require plastic surgery and skin grafts. Firefighters carried Merle, then eighty-nine, from her bedroom—because of her Alzheimer's, she could not comprehend the danger of the fire and smoke, and she could not flee on her own. She spent weeks in intensive care with lung damage from smoke inhalation. (It is one of Alzheimer's skewed gifts—unwanted but welcome at the same time—that Merle does not seem to remember the fiery inferno and the tremendous loss of that night.)

When Patricia took her mother home from the hospital, she was determined to keep her safe—and close at hand. Her husband, John, made room in his heart—and in his home office: he moved the rolltop desk, packed up his books, and installed a hospital bed. "My husband was just amazing. By the time I got [my mother] out of the ambulance, he had set her up in his old office, in a room right by the kitchen so she could be close to us and we could watch her all the time and let her feel supported," Patricia says in a telephone interview.[41] "He said, 'Everything that is good in my life I owe to this great and wonderful woman. I would do anything to give her a gentle closing on her book of life.'"

Patricia concedes that caring for a parent with Alzheimer's at home is not for everyone. But she reflects on her experience in the Peace Corps in Ethiopia, on cultures with a different view of aging, and says, "We're doing this out of love. We can make this happen. It takes time and sometimes it's start and stop, but you have to stay with it because you need to keep your goal in mind: She is going to do better at home."

While her lungs recovered, Merle needed a feeding tube to sustain her. And in order to care for her mother at home, Patricia needed to work with a local doctor. "We farm out in the Delta. There is an old country doctor who is pushing eighty. . . . [Y]ou need to have a physician who will take responsibility, and he agreed. He made house calls, and did just what doctors need to do to reassure the family, because it was touch and go the first month or so," Patricia says. "When things got sketchy sometimes, he would come. We were giving her the breathing treatments [for her smoke-damaged lungs]. You can learn how to do all these things."

Alzheimer's patients often die because they lose the ability to swallow. Like many, Merle had a feeding tube and a liquid diet. But the tube and the thickened liquid that was pumped in daily bore little resemblance to the fruits of Merle's past prowess in the kitchen, and did little to satisfy her love of a home-cooked meal. "I got her home, and we were working with the feeding tube and I thought, 'The poor darling,'" Patricia says. "Because every time you swallow, it's like somebody sticking a pencil down your throat." She called the family practitioner and told him she was going to remove the feeding tube. "I knew she was going to be able to keep swallowing. She loves to eat, I'm a good cook and I know her recipes. I know we can do this." By the time the doctor arrived, Patricia had removed the feeding tube—and watched as her mother "lit up like a candle."

By spring of 2008—less than three months after the fire—Merle was sitting in a wheelchair at the family dining table, eating Easter dinner. "She was just in love with that food, she picked up her fork, and she was eating it by herself," Patricia says. The next weekend was Patricia's birthday celebration at the family ranch, so the Garamendi family experimented. They had salvaged Merle's Cadillac after the fire, and at the outdoor barbecue, they eased her into the sumptuous seat of the old car. "We got her into the car and she felt like a queen," Patricia says now. "She was comfortable because she knew that car. We drove her up to the barn, and she came in waving like Queen Elizabeth, waving to all the grandkids." When the children began batting around balloons, Patricia noticed a flash of recognition in her mother. Merle "started putting her hands up like she wanted to be a volleyball player. And she started batting balloons back and forth with the kids."

Patricia fully acknowledges that she is blessed with the resources that allow her to keep her mother at home. And she is aware of the potential guilt factor when speaking with friends who want advice on their own parents. Her answer: There is no single model that fits every family. The course of the disease and the profile of the caregivers all factor in to the long-term plan for care of an Alzheimer's patient. And sometimes an adult day program or a long-term care facility is needed.

Her message, however, is that there is joy to be had—and often more joy than difficulty. She makes a point to meet her mother where she is, to suspend her expectations and embrace her in the present moment.

"When the grandchildren come to visit—and I have nine grandchildren under the age of nine—they play babies with her," Patricia says. "She has her babies [dolls] and they have their babies. They play back and forth, they crawl in bed with her and they read stories to her. I think of my friends who are so devoted to their parents, they'll go to the nursing home every evening to have dinner. I get to go home and be with Mom. We watch television, we watch movies. She loves DVDs like *High Society*; she loves Grace Kelly. The kids watch musicals with her, the familiar things, over and over again."

Patricia, who has raised six children, compares life with her mother to life with a new baby. It is an apt description, since Alzheimer's seems to send the brain reeling backward, attacking higher functions first. "It's finding joy in the event that is happening at that particular moment. She has her routines. In the beginning, we were working a lot with puzzles, but that was kind of a strain for her. Now we look at albums and pictures. She has all of her meals at the dining table, which is important for a sense of togetherness and properness. We had her ninetieth birthday up at the ranch, and had all of her relatives and her recipes, and a reunion with her ninety-three-year-old sister. Even though it was a barbecue, I put her in her gown and took her out in her wheelchair to watch the performers. She knew exactly what was going on."

Peter Yarrow of the folk group Peter, Paul and Mary sang at the barbecue, and the song "Leaving on a Jet Plane" was fraught with symbolism. "Because," Patricia says, "there's a whole other meaning to that song. 'My bags are packed, I'm ready to go. Kiss me and say goodbye.' It was very special because many of the relatives never will see her again. But who knows? She's quite a miracle."

What would Patricia recommend in terms of healthcare reform? What would she change about her mother's care? "We need earlier diagnosis," she says emphatically. "I think that if we had been able to diagnose Mom earlier and started her on a good combination of drugs earlier, it could have given her more quality of life. Prevention is also so important." She hopes to see a revolution in Alzheimer's care, much like the hospice movement altered the American medical establishment's treatment of death. "We've come a long way with hospice care. My younger sister died of diabetes fifteen years ago. [The medical authorities] said, 'You can't take her home; she needs to stay in the hospital.' Now it's OK to have hospice care. It's OK to have someone pass on with their family around them. All of these extraordinary measures that we do in the hospital for one more day, for one more week. We're denying that person the dignity and the joy of being surrounded by prayer and by family, snuggled up in their own beds. It's a great model for the future of Alzheimer's care. People are very hungry to do the right thing. More education is needed so that caregivers and families know what all their options are."

NOTES

1. W. Cornejo et al., "Descripción de una familia con demencia pre-senil tipo Alzheimer," *Acta Med Colombiana* 12 (1987): 55–61.

2. Because everyone with the mutant gene shares a common ancestor, Faviola's husband is most likely a distant cousin. Both her family and her husband's family come from the same small village. Like many people around the world from tiny isolated places, it is not always possible to avoid marriage between distant cousins. I was once asked by a gentleman from one of the pueblos where the Alzheimer families live whether I would counsel them against marrying their cousins, and I said yes I would. The gentleman replied, "Then who should we marry? Nearly everyone I know where I live is a cousin."

3. R. F. Clark et al., Alzheimer's Disease Collaborative Group, "The Structure of the Presenilin 1 (S182) Gene and Identification of Six Novel Mutations in Early Onset AD Families," *Nature Genetics* 11 (1995): 219–22.

4. Julie Noonan Lawson, Testimony before the Bipartisan Congressional Task Force on Alzheimer's Disease, May 3, 2005, http://www.alz.org/join_the _cause_julie_noonan_lawson_50305.asp.

5. Ibid.

6. Julie Noonan Lawson, personal interview with Ellen Clegg, October 2008.

7. Ibid.

8. Ibid.

9. Ronald Reagan letter about Alzheimer's diagnosis, November 5, 1994, "Primary Sources," PBS, http://www.pbs.org/wgbh/amex/presidents/40 _reagan/psources/ps_alzheimers.html.

10. Leslie Feldman, telephone interview with Ellen Clegg, January 2009.

11. Ronald Reagan, "Farewell Address to the Nation," January 11, 1989, http://www.ronaldreagan.com/sp_21.html.

12. Terence Smith, "Stealing Minds," *NewsHour with Jim Lehrer*, June 8, 2004, http://www.pbs.org/newshour/bb/remember/jan-june04/minds_06-08 .html.

13. David Shenk, *The Forgetting, Alzheimer's: Portrait of an Epidemic* (New York: Anchor Books, 2003), p. 19.

14. Douglas Brinkley, ed., *The Reagan Diaries*, abridged ed., The Ronald Reagan Presidential Library Foundation (New York: HarperCollins, 2007), p. 13.

15. Ibid.

16. Ibid., p. 14.

17. Ibid., p. 17.

18. Edmund Morris, *Dutch: A Memoir of Ronald Reagan* (New York: Random House, 1999), p. 629.

19. Nicholas Wapshott, "Ronald Reagan and Margaret Thatcher, A Political Marriage," Sentinel, 2008, pp. 267–68.

20. Morris, *Dutch*, pp. 655–56.

21. Feldman, telephone interview with Ellen Clegg, January 2009.

22. Biography, Margaret Thatcher Foundation, http://www.margaret thatcher.org/essential/biography.asp#ess87–90.

23. Thatcher letter to Reagan upon inaugural, Margaret Thatcher Foundation, Reagan Library: NSA Head of State File (Box 35), http://www .margaretthatcher.org/archive/displaydocument.asp?docid=109292.

24. Reagan cable to Thatcher about upcoming visit, Margaret Thatcher Foundation, Reagan Library: NSA head of State File (Thatcher: Cables [1] Box 34).

25. Thatcher's February 25, 1981, visit to Washington, Margaret Thatcher Foundation, Sir Nicholas Henderson diary, Wednesday, February 25, 1981.

26. Stanislao Pugliese, telephone interview with Ellen Clegg, January 2009.

27. Carol Thatcher, "I Always Thought of Mum as Being 100% Cast-Iron Damage Proof," *Daily Mail*, August 23, 2008, http://www.dailymail.co.uk/femail/article-1048540/Carol-Thatcher-I-thought-Mum-100-cast-iron-damage -proof.html.

28. Ibid.

29. Ibid.

30. Ibid.

31. Ibid.

32. Ibid.

33. Ibid.

34. Amanda Platell, "Too Soon and In Too Much Detail: Why I'm Saddened by Carol Thatcher's Tell-All Book on Her Mother's Dementia," *Daily Mail*, August 26, 2008, http://www.dailymail.co.uk/femail/article-1048858/ Too-soon-far-Why-Im-saddened-Carol-Thatchers-tell-book-mothers -dementia.html.

35. Ibid.

36. Pugliese, telephone interview with Ellen Clegg, January 2009.

37. Jane Gross, "The New Old Age," *New York Times*, September 2, 2008, http://newoldage.blogs.nytimes.com/2008/09/02/margaret-thatchers -open-secret/.

38. Alexander Chancellor, "Carol Thatcher Was Rebuked for Revealing Her Mother Had Dementia, but It Is Nothing to Be Ashamed Of," *Guardian*, September 19, 2008, http://www.guardian.co.uk/commentisfree/2008/sep/19/features.comment.

39. Patricia Garamendi, "Mama, the Grandest Lady," *care ADvantage*, Summer 2007, pp. 12–13.

40. Patricia Garamendi, speech given at the Alzheimer's Foundation of America, 3rd National Concepts in Care Conference, San Francisco, September 18, 2008.

41. Patricia Garamendi, telephone interview with Ellen Clegg, January 2009.

2

WHY WE NEED
NEIGHBORHOOD COGNITIVE SHOPS

The brain is wider than the sky,
For, put them side by side,
The one the other will include
With ease, and you beside.

The brain is deeper than the sea,
For, hold them, blue to blue,
The one the other will absorb,
As sponges, buckets do.

The brain is just the weight of God,
For, lift them, pound for pound,
And they will differ, if they do,
As syllable from sound.
—EMILY DICKINSON, "THE BRAIN IS WIDER THAN THE SKY"

NOWHERE TO TURN

The approach taken in Colombia, with its rich skein of family kinship, to the scourge of Alzheimer's that has haunted generations is not necessarily a solution for wealthier nations. But the story unfolding in small barrios holds lessons, nevertheless, and shows what is missing in Alzheimer's care in the United States.

Many pieces to the puzzle of Alzheimer's are missing, and the pieces we do have are scattered far and wide. Whether an individual already has some degree of dementia or is mentally sharp but feels the looming risk of dementia as she ages, the programs and services she needs reside in separate silos. Sustaining cognitive health in our elderly population is particularly challenging because it requires the coordination of professionals from a wide variety of disciplines that are not usually found in any single location. Trekking from doctor's office to clinic to social worker in an attempt to piece together the expertise needed for a cognitive health program can be exhausting for patients and their families. While centers with state-of-the-art approaches to eye care, dental care, and physical fitness are thriving, nowhere do we have centers that focus on cognition. Such comprehensive centers simply do not exist.

Needs cannot be met by busy and oversubscribed local physicians, particularly those who see numerous patients during a workday and must bill Medicare for specific services in order to be reimbursed. Jan Thorgaard, a retired computer programmer in the upper Midwest, still recalls the brusque treatment she received when she was seeking a diagnosis for her husband, Harold. Married forty-two years to her best friend from high school, Jan was winding down her career and looking forward to a season of relaxation and travel with her husband, who was ready to shutter his appliance repair business. For two sixty-somethings raised on farms, the world beckoned. But Harold had begun forgetting. Used to traveling from town to town for his job, he could not keep his itinerary straight. He would trail off midsentence in conversation, unsure of the right words. For a while, it seemed like a normal part of aging. And after so many years together, Jan had no trouble finishing Harold's sentences for him. Finally, Jan says, Harold reached the point of frustration and decided to get checked out by a local physician.

"He got to the point where he had to find out what was happening to him. So he went to see the doctor to get tests done," she says. Jan, who projects calm and wisdom, was shocked at what happened next: the doctor appeared in the examining room, announced that Harold had Alzheimer's, and walked out. That was the abrupt beginning of a terrifying new phase of life together. "He never came back. It was terrible. He could have said something human, or handed us some information, or anything, really. We just kind of looked at each other and then went home and cried."[1]

While Jan and Harold's experience might seem extreme, the fact is that physicians are boxed in. The Medicare system, which pays physicians a fee for each service rendered, is not set up to handle a disease like Alzheimer's, which can affect patients for years and years. "The

Medicare Fee-for-Service system, which covers more than 80 percent of Medicare enrollees, was designed to address acute conditions and rewards providers for a high volume of in-office services. This reimbursement policy effectively discourages the between-visit care and support most valuable to people with dementia and their family caregivers," according to a report issued in spring of 2009 by the bipartisan Alzheimer's Study Group, cochaired by former congressman Newt Gingrich and former senator Bob Kerrey. The report, given the ambitious title "A National Alzheimer's Strategic Plan," elaborated: "There are interventions proven to increase quality of life for people with dementia while optimizing their healthcare utilization. Yet, many of the most promising interventions—including community-based psychosocial interventions and caregiver counseling programs—are not covered by Medicare Fee-for-Service."[2]

And not all needs are being met by the Alzheimer's Disease Research Centers (ADRCs), a network of researchers funded by the National Institute on Aging at twenty-nine major medical centers across the United States. Although researchers at these centers are working to translate the latest research advances into improvements in care for patients, such centers are often in elite teaching hospitals in urban areas, and treatment reaches only a rarefied slice of the population. The centers, based on excellent medical campuses like the Feinberg School of Medicine at Northwestern University in Chicago, conduct research and train scientists and healthcare providers.[3]

Although the National Institute on Aging notes that the ADRCs act as a network to share new ideas and research results, they tend to cover only a fraction of what patients with cognitive problems want to know. While some centers have satellite clinics that offer services and research opportunities in underserved, rural, and minority communities, the number of centers remains far too insignificant. Even in the halls of some of the most storied teaching hospitals in the United States, services can be fragmented, requiring patients to navigate a maze of buildings spread over a large medical campus. A look at the menu of services offered by one such center, the Alzheimer Disease Research Center at the University of Pittsburgh, shows that it offers comprehensive diagnostic evaluations for patients—including neuropsychological testing of memory, language, judgment, and other cognitive abilities. It also allows patients to participate in clinical trials. But patients and their families must get referrals to physicians, community social service agencies, transportation services, adult daycare, support groups, and other programs that cannot be found in one place.[4]

Most ADRCs are not even aware of these shortfalls in their services because they do not ask patients about their satisfaction with the program. Instead, their success depends on reviews from members of the twenty-nine ADRCs in the network. On the one hand, we are left with a system that does little to meet many of the needs of Alzheimer patients. On the other hand, local physicians are overburdened, often lack the necessary expertise or interest in the problem, and do not have available any of the nonphysician services required by Alzheimer patients. Most distressing is that while it is widely acknowledged that prevention is the most effective way to reduce the incidence of the disease, centers that focus on sustaining cognitive health in middle-aged and elderly people are not even on the drawing board. One might go so far as to say that the medical system, with its emphasis on the fifteen-minute office visit, its complex insurance schemes, and most important, a reimbursement system that pays doctors only for treating a disease, not preventing a disease, is actually an obstacle to implementing prevention and achieving lifelong cognitive health.

The bipartisan Alzheimer's Study Group recommends expanding and enhancing the network of Alzheimer's Disease Research Centers. "The existing . . . [centers] should serve as foundation to create centers like the National Cancer Institute's Comprehensive Care Centers. These centers would incorporate and support efforts focused on establishing a national registry for longitudinal studies, qualifying biomarkers, developing therapies, conducting research on models of care, carrying out community-based research and education, and training and retaining new investigators." In fact, the study group stresses integration, bringing together everything from basic research through delivery of care. The group's report also emphasizes the need for geographic sweep in order to open up access for those who live in underserved areas. "It may also be advisable to pilot and refine a single comprehensive center and then use this experience in a subsequent expansion of the Comprehensive Alzheimer's Disease Centers infrastructure."[5] The study group repeatedly calls for new funding to avoid diluting current research efforts.

After a patient undergoes a battery of medical tests and receives a diagnosis of Alzheimer's disease, much goes unsaid. Typically, what the physician does not say is that life expectancy from the time of diagnosis averages ten years—long years during which the medical system often abandons the patient. Many of the issues that arise in the decade after diagnosis are not medical and are best handled by caregivers who are not doctors—social workers and occupational or physical therapists are among the professionals most frequently needed. No comprehensive approach to this long, insidious period of decline exists. Physicians are left with the option of prescribing one or two FDA-approved drugs that offer minimal benefit.

Marcel Agüeros is an accomplished professional, yet he often feels daunted by the dense bureaucracy he must navigate to secure fragmented care for his father, New York poet Jack Agüeros. When Alzheimer's disease began to still the voice of Jack Agüeros, known for vivid descriptions of Puerto Rican culture and experience in New York City, Marcel moved back home to help. "The primary weight for a long time, and the only weight, was on my sister, because I was in graduate school in Seattle when my father first started to display signs that things were not quite right. I was not directly involved in day-to-day stuff. I would come back occasionally," Marcel says. During one visit, Marcel enrolled his father at the Veterans Administration hospital because he didn't have any health insurance. "My sister took the brunt of it. To be honest, I was skeptical. She was telling me that my dad was doing poorly and that certain things were happening. I didn't really believe—or want to believe—that things were as bad as she was saying."[6]

Marcel recalls a precise moment, a reckoning, with his father's deteriorating condition: One Christmas, he arrived in New York from Seattle to find a pile of Jack's bills that had not been paid. It was then he realized that his father "just couldn't do it anymore and that I had to take that responsibility."

Natalia Agüeros lives next door to her father, and Marcel is now a National Science Foundation astronomy and astrophysics fellow at Columbia University, an academic job with some flexibility that allows him time for forays into New York's tangled social services network. Marcel has the time needed to fill out thick sheaves of forms for Medicaid, and hours and hours to stand in line to apply for food stamps for his father. Although Marcel has certainly mastered complexity in his professional life—his research is titled "A Multiwavelength Study of the Galactic Plane and of its Stellar Remnants"—he laughs as he admits to being flummoxed by the twists and turns of Medicaid regulations.

"I certainly have some of the skills required to fill out the paperwork, although not all of them. I'm not sure who has all of them. It was very hard in my first year and a half," Marcel says. "I felt like I was doing two or three jobs at the same time. I was trying to balance my own career after transitioning into this new job, and dealing with my dad, and trying to fix my personal life. It was just really, really messy. It's not like I'm asking for sympathy, but I think that getting the home care, getting Medicaid approved, was transformative because I don't worry about my dad on a daily basis anymore. I don't worry that he is wandering the building or that he is not eating or that he hasn't showered. There are a whole set of concerns that I don't have anymore."

Marcel is coming to terms with the many hours of care needed to keep his father at home. "One of the things you realize is that the more hours you cover in a day, the more remaining hours there are. We need more hours for him; that is clearly becoming the case." When emergencies happen, either Marcel or Natalia must cancel plans and juggle schedules to fill the gaps. Marcel recalls a particular week, just before the Medicaid application came through, when his sister and his father were both sick. He dropped everything and took the twenty-minute subway ride from his home on the Upper West Side to his father's apartment to help. During the holidays, he and his sister split up—one attends family gatherings (their mother lives in Europe) and the other tends to their father. He recalls waiting in line for three hours at the food stamp office and never getting to the right person—and not having time to return. Coincidentally, one of Jack's sonnets ruminates on the stultifying experience of standing in line for benefits at an unemployment office:

Sonnet Substantially Like the Words of Fulano Rodriguez
One Position Ahead of Me On the Unemployment Line

It happens to me all the time—business
Goes up and down but I'm the yo-yo spun
Into the high speed trick called sleeping
Such as I am fast standing in this line now.
Maybe I am also a top; they too sleep
While standing, tightly twirling in place.
I wish I could step out and listen for
The sort of music that I must make.
But this is where the state celebrates its sport.
From cushioned chairs the agents turn your ample
Time against you through a box of lines.
Your string is both your leash and lash.
The faster you spin, the stiller you look.
There's something to learn in that, but what?

—Jack Agüeros,
from *Correspondence between the Stonehaulers* (1991)[7]

What would ideal care look like? Marcel takes a moment for the broad view: It is clear, he says, that Alzheimer's disease does not get the kind of attention it needs. "I'm not interested into getting into debates about which diseases are more horrible or more deserving of funding or attention," he says. "It's a demographic time bomb. Because we don't talk about aging or the elderly or death very much at all in this country, I think as a society we're largely ignorant of the toll this is taking on caregivers and families."

Care is fragmented, he notes, splintered among city and federal agencies and insurers with differing regulations. "You have to go to different places for different aspects of the care. That does make it incredibly difficult. Certainly something that is more integrated would be really useful. I think the most important thing for me is that I was able to join an Alzheimer's support group very early on. I think the Alzheimer's Association chapter here in New York does a really nice job of trying to coordinate these efforts and help you navigate the legal, the financial, and the emotional waters."

But the arc of Alzheimer's is harrowing, with multiple layers of loss. "I think that's the part that makes it such a horrible disease. You've lost someone but they're still with you, so you're in a permanent state of mourning." His father is still happy and healthy, Marcel says, and he wants him around for a long time. "But right now, it just seems like suffering for suffering's sake."

THE NEIGHBORHOOD COGNITIVE SHOP

Because the incidence of Alzheimer's disease is so high in the elderly population, some form of prevention is an important part of a health program. But patients and families are left to figure out on their own the most effective preventive measures because physicians are not reimbursed for spending time with an at-risk individual. One solution to this problem is to enhance lifelong cognitive health nationally through the placement of "cognitive shops" in our communities. In Santa Barbara we have established a pilot site for the delivery of cognitive services to the community called the Center for Cognitive Fitness and Innovative Therapies (CFIT). Within a space of about twenty-five hundred square feet, a small staff can provide nearly all of the services needed for Alzheimer's disease prevention and guide the care of those with mild or moderate disease.

The program begins by assessing the two overarching areas where prevention can make a difference: medical risk factors and lifestyle risk factors. Obtaining a data set for each individual at the center, called the *evaluation*, is the first step. A care coordinator collects the information. Once the data have been collected, a program for cognitive health is devised and presented to the client at a team meeting with members of the CFIT staff and the client's family. The implementation of the program, called the *intervention*, is the second step.

The first data sought in the center concern the major medical risks for dementia: blood pressure, lipid profile, and blood glucose. All are easily measured values that affect an individual's lifelong risk for cognitive decline. In fact, these three simple values are the strongest known risk factors for dementia, other than aging itself. These risks are probably familiar to most people because they are also risk factors for cardiovascular disease. The overlap between risk factors for dementia and cardiovascular illness is telling; the brain is simply an organ in the body, and, like any other organ, it requires a good blood supply. Anything that affects cardiovascular health is likely to affect the brain.

Abnormalities in any or all of these measurements are treatable. These measurements are routine for primary-care doctors, but many people do not regularly visit their primary-care doctor, and if they do, vigilance about blood pressure control or how to implement healthy lifestyle changes may be beyond what a busy medical doctor can accomplish within a brief office visit once a year. By the time a patient sees a neurologist, his or her needs have usually changed from prevention to treatment, and in a specialty setting, the more routine medical inquiries concerning a healthy lifestyle are often overlooked. Certainly, cognitive health does not respect the boundaries set up around neurological practices with their focus on neurological disease, so our first step is general medical health, particularly those factors that affect cognition. It is clear that nowhere in medicine have we created sites where we can optimize the advance measures we take to reduce the incidence of dementia.

Once the baseline medical information is in place, data collection shifts to learning about the individual's lifestyle. Here, once again, the information needed is not extensive and is based on research that has identified factors that favor lifelong cognitive health. Those factors are exercise, diet, social connections, reduction of chronic stress, and cognitive challenges. Standardized formats built out from existing electronic medical programs allow entry of exercise and dietary information. A simple test for assessing social support is the International Support Evaluation List (ISEL) questionnaire. This simple test is made up of a list of forty statements designed to probe the perceived availability of social resources, from having someone with whom to talk about problems, to having people with whom to do things. Half of the questions are positive statements about social relationships (for example, "If I were sick, I could easily find someone to help me with my daily chores"); the other half are negative statements (such as, "I feel that there is no one with whom I can share my most private worries and fears"). Respondents are asked to indicate whether each statement is "probably true" or "probably false." The ISEL is scored by counting the number of responses indicating support.[8]

A useful measurement scale of chronic stress is the Holmes-Rahe Social Readjustment Rating Scale, which measures life changes.[9] This five-minute questionnaire lists a series of stressors that may have occurred in an individual's life over the past two years, ranked according to severity. Each stressor is assigned a score measured in "life crisis units"; the most severe stressors are death of a spouse (100 units), followed by divorce (73 units) and marital separation (65 units). Among the lowest-ranking stressors—but a stressor nevertheless—is taking a vacation, which comes in at 13 life crisis units. There is no standardized format for obtaining baseline information about the cognitive challenges an individual faces; however, simply entering a person's occupation, hobbies, life goals, and how he spends time can offer a reasonable subjective assessment and serve as the basis for the design of interventions. In some cases, these questions may identify areas related to spiritual concerns or end-of-life issues that will need in-depth attention.

After the data collection, all clients undergo baseline neuropsychological testing performed by a trained assistant. Having a baseline score of an individual's cognitive performance is important in order to assess whether any future issues that crop up in the area of thinking and memory represent a real decline.

This approach to assessment minimizes expenses related to physician time, compared to the current system. Current practice places the physician on the front line to deal with all of the patient's issues, using information gathered by having the patient fill out a thick sheaf of forms. The frequent duplication of questions on these forms can be maddening and with the physician as the only backstop for the myriad of problems listed many patient complaints get ignored.

All data are entered into a dynamic electronic medical record (EMR) designed to flag the medical and lifestyle factors that require attention. One of the benefits of an EMR is improved communication—after all, any record of cognitive health should not be isolated from a patient's other medical records. In the future, the EMR of cognitive health should be integrated with other computerized medical records. Extracting the necessary data from a voluminous patient history is time consuming. A computer program that can search a patient's history is badly needed in order to extract critical notes and lab reports relevant to a specific problem. Electronic medical records should also be accessible online to the patient and perhaps linked to reliable information about each item on the patient problem list.

After the evaluation phase is complete, the team holds a review meeting for the client and the client's family. The goal is to present a personalized program and develop a common purpose among the key individuals who will track the patient's progress. The members of the team at the review are the care coordinator; a physician, usually an internist; and the Navigator, who is expert at sifting good information from bad on the Web, and who keeps up with the latest online sources for scientific and medical developments. The Navigator is central to the local cognitive shop. She is not a doctor. Instead, she knows how to obtain information on a broad range of topics related to cognition. The Navigator is the connection between vast realms of specialized knowledge and people in the community.

The team meeting takes place around a table with the client and family members. Some family members may not be physically in the room but are instead connected remotely through videoconferencing. In some cases, the team may identify the need for further medical treatment, such as improved blood pressure control. In other cases—such as when a family history suggests some inheritable risk—the client may want a more detailed genetic analysis of her DNA. The Navigator projects data and Web-based points of information on the wall. For example, an individual who has just been diagnosed with the earliest stages of Alzheimer's disease may want to know what research programs are available. The Navigator can project regional and national research sites, experimental medications, and a list of entry criteria. Using this information, a directed search by the Navigator can quickly cut through the overwhelming amount of information on the Web, do data triage, and tell the person about the experimental medication being offered. Entry into most research programs is biased in favor of the facility at which the person happens to show up for care. Someone who goes to an Alzheimer center at a major university will be referred to those clinical trials going on at that university and will not be told about any other trials. Someone who goes to a local physician who has some connection to a clinical trial—a rare circumstance—will be referred to the trial the physician is being paid to conduct and will not be told about any other trials. The Navigator, who is not associated with any clinical trial, can present an overview of all current research. In essence the Navigator is a purveyor of information: someone who is there to answer questions. Because no single individual can be expected to have encyclopedic knowledge about such a rapidly changing subject, the Navigator can be thought of as a human search engine who works with clients to get the best possible information. The absence of any such position in the medical field is currently a major source of patient frustration.

Based on the individual data, the team arrives at a personalized treatment program and any further evaluation that may be needed. To many, the word *personalized* evokes elite images: customized, hand holding, one-on-one, concierge medicine, boutique medicine. Most of all, it seems to be another way of saying "expensive." But the association between personalized medicine and luxury medicine needs to be broken. If medical treatment is more individualized, many facets of care delivery that are ineffective will be eliminated. Getting away from the one-size-fits-all philosophy will reduce side effects and redundant services. Key to making personalized medicine available to many is an efficient flow of the data stream that marks individual differences in patient histories, in their reaction to medications, in their lifestyles, and in their genetics. The cognitive shop has established exactly what information must enter the data stream to provide a personalized program. Thus, a "smart" data stream in conjunction with services related to cognition all located at a single site is likely to become a highly cost-effective way to supplant a problem that is now generally ignored or approached in a highly fragmented manner.

Based on the evaluation, the team defines an implementation program. The recommended program for most clients will include exercise, diet, stress reduction, and cognitive challenges. The recommended mix has to fit with the individual's lifestyle, and it must be practical and medically within the limits of what the client can do. Most challenging is adherence to the regimen. Lack of adherence to any medical program—even taking a daily medication—is one of the main reasons for treatment failure. By far the most effective way to persuade people to change their behavior is through social pressure. The evidence for these effects is overwhelming, and the power of social networks in affecting healthy behaviors is only just beginning to be explored (see chapter 9). Therefore, a place where people go for prevention of cognitive impairment is more likely to be effective than a program that requires the individual to do activities in his home. Group participation helps increase adherence and enjoyment in doing activities that might be tedious if done solo.

COMMUNITY ACCEPTANCE OF COGNITIVE CENTERS AND PHYSICIAN REFERRAL PATTERNS

Cognitive centers service two demographics: healthy elders and those with dementia. The healthy elder who would like to optimize every measure possible for lifelong cognitive health is well suited for the services provided by a cognitive shop. Because prevention is the number one means we have to make an impact on dementia, healthy elders are a primary target group. However, the cognitive shop cannot ignore those individuals already diagnosed with cognitive impairment who require attention during the long period of decline after their diagnosis—the time when the existing medical system fails.

CFIT grades clients into three tiers: those who are cognitively intact, those with minimal cognitive impairment or very early stage Alzheimer's disease, and those with frank dementia. For those individuals in the most severely affected category, CFIT does not offer services on site, instead offering consultations and connections to services in the community through a caretaker. Assisted living facilities provide one approach for elders who need help caring for themselves. However, the greatest gap is in the treatment of those at risk for dementia, and that includes a very large number of people.

The ideal entry point to a cognitive center comes after the client has made contact with a community physician. Community-based cognitive centers are intended to provide added value to existing physician services by reducing the burden on doctors after they have completed an initial, routine medical workup. The cognitive center will then be in contact with the physician to offer its recommendations for next steps, and opinions on whether those next steps should be implemented by the physician or through the center. In this manner, cognitive centers can grow in communities without upsetting the economic structure among physicians who are already practicing. The presence of a cognitive shop offering all services in one location is far more efficient than the convoluted path between far-flung ancillary services and far more economical than placing the physician as the centerpiece. Currently, primary-care doctors tend to send the problem of dementia to an expensive specialist such as a neurologist, and after waiting months to see the specialist, the patient is often simply passed back to the primary-care doctor.

A recent audit of neurologists revealed that 62 percent of patients had undergone a clinical investigation for dementia before being seen by the neurologist. Often, the primary-care doctor had ordered the appropriate tests, and in more than a third of the cases the primary-care doctor had initiated an appropriate treatment using drugs. The primary-care doctor felt that the referral was necessary, and in many cases, even neurologists made referrals to other neurologists with a subspecialty interest in dementia. Only a relatively small subset of neurologists welcome Alzheimer patients because the dementia field is highly specialized and lacks procedures that have higher reimbursements. With such a small group of subspecialists directing their attention to Alzheimer's disease, the numbers of such physicians are completely inadequate to care for the aging population.

About three-quarters of the primary-care referrals audited did not present complicated behavioral problems or diagnostic puzzles. Thus, most of the cases were not challenging—and yet the referring doctors were uncomfortable handling these cases themselves. Despite the relative competence of primary-care doctors in handling cases of dementia, there was one glaring omission: the primary physicians frequently ordered expensive brain-imaging procedures such as CT and MRI scans, but failed to administer the mini–mental status exam (MMSE), a basic, twenty-minute questionnaire widely used as a standard for the diagnosis of dementia. Mental status testing is one of the most low-tech tests in all of medicine—and it was often missing. As a result, primary-care doctors in the study referred patients for dementia testing when in fact 6 percent had no cognitive impairment and 15 percent had only mild impairment and did not qualify for the diagnosis of dementia.[10]

The leap to expensive tests—as seen here by the overuse of brain imaging without first performing a simple pencil-and-paper mental status test—is a major contributor to high medical costs. As noted in a report by the Congressional Budget Office, the aging of the US population contributes less to health expenditure growth than do increases in the volume of care per patient.[11] Costly interventions and the introduction of expensive new diagnostic tests, procedures, and other treatments have boosted costs, and elders are among the major consumers of these expensive procedures and tests. Community-based cognitive centers can help stem the tide of overutilization of these expensive services. For example, when baseline neuropsychological data are on file and a client arrives complaining of memory loss, the knee-jerk reaction to schedule an MRI scan may be avoided in many cases because the center can document that no memory decline has occurred. Something else might explain the patient's complaint. If a recent MRI is on file, caregivers in cognitive centers—where an electronic medical record is de rigeur and where the emphasis is on obtaining the existing record and coordinating care—are less likely to repeat an expensive test.

ACHIEVING LIFELONG BRAIN HEALTH

Having friends is a strong predictor of lifelong health, even into old age. Part of successful aging seems to be having friends. How can the cognitive shop help elders, as they become increasingly isolated, sustain friendships? As such centers are developed—based on a model of care similar to that offered at CFIT—they will use data collected in patient interviews to enhance interconnections by building social networks among elders in the community. These networks will be built by asking clients to provide the names of ten close friends and, as the client base grows, the interconnections among the population served by the center will help stave off the isolation that is so common among elders. An elder who needed help with an errand, or just a friendly ear on the telephone, could check the social network to find someone to help and to facilitate friendships that come much more easily for younger people.

Establishing life goals during the retirement years is critical for lifelong brain health. Yet raising such questions with one's physician almost sounds ludicrous. People often turn to a church group or a community center, but involvement in such groups is not realistic for everyone. So where can one turn for an informed discussion, the way a student might discuss career options with a high school guidance counselor? Sometimes the only person left with whom an individual can have a frank discussion about life's options as an elder is his attorney, accountant, or even a tax preparer. Overlooked are the many people who can offer substantive suggestions. Libraries, for example, have expanded their role in the Internet age, providing public computers so anyone can get online. Perhaps their role could evolve further, functioning, in part, as a cognitive center where information is readily available on healthy aging. Librarians could serve as Navigators who can guide wandering elders toward late-life goals. The skills and resources of our libraries are also the domain of cognitive shops.

As the Web, and Navigators using the Web, increasingly come to the service of those with memory impairment, even healthy elders might find some benefit from the array of tools offered in cognitive shops. CFIT includes a memory archive. Undergraduate students are recruited to film and edit interviews with clients who may have concerns about their future ability to communicate their life stories to their children, grandchildren, and great-grandchildren. These recordings can provide a way for elders to express their wishes about life-sustaining measures, should they be needed. This recorded story might someday help a caretaker hired to provide total care to a person she never met as a vibrant personality, who now, with little ability to communicate, seems only to inhabit his body. Watching a video that shows a fully functioning human being with his own speaking style, sense of humor, and facial expressions will likely improve the care given by aides and other hired strangers who come along to tend to the patient. We know very well that attachments are built between people through empathy—by watching the emotions of others and feeling that same emotion in ourselves. A chronicle of one's life is one way to build empathy for the cognitively debilitated. With a recording in hand, it's only a short step to upload a memoir to YouTube and post it as an interactive Internet link on a social networking site like Facebook in order to keep an archive that can be shared with others.

CFIT works with Kate Carter of LifeChronicles to memorialize people's stories. Here is how Kate describes her work on her Web site: "Through videotaping individuals and families across the country, LifeChronicles strives to preserve the memory and essence of individuals, to tell the stories that could have gone untold and to solidify the bonds between people. With the help of our youth volunteers, LifeChronicles has served over 400 families and has found a need for our video-recordings in a variety of similar situations."[12]

FINDING SUPPORT IN THE COMMUNITY

One key element for helping elders, particularly those with dementia, find the support they need can be found in an existing method, known as time banking.[13] Here is how the programs work: For every hour an individual spends doing something for someone in her community, she earns one time dollar. Then she has a time dollar to spend on having someone do something for her. It's that simple, but it also has profound effects. Time banks change neighborhoods and whole communities. Time banking is a social change movement in twenty-two countries and on six continents. The center will provide a platform for the formation of time-banking communities.

Time banking works at the grass roots of American life. Participants use time bank software to make a list of services they need—carpooling for children or respite care for an elderly relative or help with grocery shopping. Participants then look at a list of people offering services, and can either e-mail directly or work through the community agency coordinating the time bank. (A computer is not essential. Some agencies coordinate tasks and services by phone, according to the Web site www.timebanks.org .) The system is used by charitable agencies all over the United States, and by volunteer groups of concerned neighbors who band together to help with lawn mowing, childcare, eldercare, or even music lessons. In Massachusetts alone, there are five volunteer groups in communities as far-flung as picturesque Cape Ann on the coast and the industrial city of Lynn.

How does time banking and spending work? The Web site finds a prime example in PeopleLink, a Denver, Colorado, collaborative between Catholic Charities, Lutheran Family Services of Colorado, and Jewish Family Services of Colorado. PeopleLink, which focuses on helping elders remain independent, became interested in recruiting volunteers to help with a mutual exchange of services in 1999.

During the first year alone, according to www.timebanks.org, PeopleLink helped broker the exchange of nearly seven hundred hours of services—such as transportation to doctors' visits—for the elderly and for people with disabilities.

The Web site paints a picture of a typical exchange:

> Cale, a physically disabled woman with limited use of her hands who uses an electric wheelchair, reached a point of desperation trying to create order out of the chaos resulting from a recent move. She urgently needed to have help unpacking, for among her personal papers was critical income information that she needed to complete paperwork making it possible for her to live in her own home.
>
> Jeffi, a retired social worker and PeopleLink participant, came to her rescue, sorting out boxes and wiping down shelves on which to place their contents. After Jeffi helped her locate the important papers, she helped Cale complete the required forms.
>
> Cale plans to reciprocate by teaching people computer skills, writing articles, and editing the PeopleLink newsletter.[14]

As the medical system grows more impenetrable, a frequent conclusion is that the burden of care should shift back to the primary-care physician, a long-standing rallying cry for policymakers. But private offices—without access to staffing, educational materials, and support to meet the needs of the demented patient and the patient's family—may find it to be both difficult and an inefficient use of their time to accept these referrals. The more important question is: Where are all the primary-care doctors? In many communities, they have all but disappeared. How many graduating medical students are entering primary care? Not very many now, and the numbers are declining. In 2009 there were 2,535 family medicine residencies offered, 101 fewer than the previous year. Also in 2009, just 2,632 US medical students matched to internal medicine residency programs, compared to 3,884 in 1985.[15] And only 20 to 25 percent of residents in internal medicine ultimately choose to practice in that area, compared to 50 percent in 1998. On the other hand, interest is strong in specialties with a heavy procedural focus, such as neurosurgery, orthopedics, otolaryngology, and dermatology. Steven E. Weinberger, the senior vice president for medical education and publishing at the American College of Physicians (APC), has said, "We are witnessing a generational shift from medical careers that specialize in preventive care, diagnostic evaluation, and long-term treatment of complex and chronic diseases, to specialties and subspecialties that provide specific procedures or a very limited focus of care."[16]

It is hard to shift the burden to primary-care doctors when there is no one at the receiving end. But much of the role of a primary-care doctor in the area of cognition is as an expensive middle manager who links patients' needs with other services. So cognitive shops that bring in medical personnel only when needed to deal with the problem of dementia would ease the existing burden posed by a high number of referrals, including those between the primary-care doctor and the neurologist. In this setting the MD is not the gatekeeper; rather the MD works as part of a team devoted to cognition.

A cognitive shop in every neighborhood may not be realistic for some communities, but a virtual, online cognitive shop is possible. However, in this endeavor we must take a lesson from the newly minted personal genomic companies. Companies such as 23andMe and Navigenics offer their genetic prediction services online. The idea was that people would sign up on the Web to mail in their saliva (which is full of DNA—so you spit in a tube to get your sample), and several weeks later they would receive an analysis with information on mutations that could lead to disease. But predicting the future is a chancy game. The companies thought they would be the fortune-tellers of the genome, but once clients received the information, they often turned to their local doctors—who, unfortunately, are often not trained in genetics and are as uncomfortable with the information as the patient. The personal genome companies, as they are now structured, cannot succeed without the human interface. For cognitive shops, personal interaction will serve people best. That said, with a shift toward Web-based services and people's increasing comfort with spending time in a virtual world, we cannot ignore the potential of the online cognitive shop.

Put more succinctly, the ideal model for the future of Alzheimer's treatment will necessitate stitching together the fragmented and bureaucratic system of care that exists now. It will mean pulling together the many aspects of medical and social care—doctors, geneticists, social workers, nutritionists—and consolidating them under one roof. It will redefine the role of the physician: Rather than seeing an Alzheimer's patient in a fifteen-minute office visit and then recording a coded diagnosis in order to be reimbursed, the physician will work with a care coordinator who at CFIT is a physical therapist, but could come from any of the ancillary services, to orchestrate a sweeping program of care that draws upon the staff in a cognitive shop, and that views the patient as a human being with a rich history, not just as a set of symptoms and complaints.

NOTES

1. Jan Thorgaard (pseudonym), telephone interview with Ellen Clegg, January 2009.

2. Alzheimer's Study Group, "A National Alzheimer's Strategic Plan: The Report of the Alzheimer's Study Group," March 2009, p. 4, http://www.alz .org/documents/national/report_ASG_alzplan.pdf (accessed February 1, 2009).

3. US National Institutes of Health, National Institute on Aging, "AD Research Centers," Alzheimer's Disease Education & Referral Center, http:// www.nia.nih.gov/Alzheimers/ResearchInformation/ResearchCenters (accessed May 19, 2009).

4. University of Pittsburgh Alzheimer's Disease Research Center, http:// www.adrc.pitt.edu/contact.asp (accessed May 19, 2009).

5. Alzheimer's Study Group, "A National Alzheimer's Strategic Plan," p. 25.

6. Marcel Agüeros, telephone interview with Ellen Clegg, January 2009.

7. Copyright by Jack Agüeros; used by permission of Hanging Loose Press.

8. Sheldon Cohen et al., "Measuring the Functional Components of Social Support," in *Social Support: Theory, Research, and Application*, ed. I. G. Sarason and B. R. Sarason (The Hague: Martinus Nijhoff, 1985).

9. Thomas Holmes and Richard Rahe, "The Social Readjustment Rating Scale," *Journal of Psychosomatic Research* 11 (1967): 213–18.

10. Details on time banking may be found at TimeBanks USA, http:// www.timebanks.org (accessed February 1, 2010).

11. TimeBanks USA Member Directory, http://www.timebanks.org/ directory.htm (accessed May 27, 2009).

12. LifeChronicles, http://www.lifechronicles.org (accessed February 1, 2010).

13. T. W. Chow et al., "100 Years after Alzheimer: Contemporary Neu-

rology Practice Assessment of Referrals for Dementia," *American Journal of Alzheimer's Disease and Other Dementias* 23, no. 6 (2008): 516–27.

14. Congressional Budget Office, "Technological Change and the Growth of Health Care Spending," January 2008, http://www.cbo.gov/ftpdocs/89xx/doc8947/01-31-TechHealth.pdf (accessed May 12, 2009).

15. American College of Physicians, "Residency Match Results Demonstrate Need to Address National Primary Care Workforce Goals," *ACP News*, March 19, 2009, http://www.acponline.org/pressroom/09_match.htm (accessed August 31, 2009).

16. Steven E. Weinberger, quoted in American College of Physicians, "Residency Match Results."

3

UNDERSTANDING THE BASICS

Where We Are, How We Got Here

And surely it is a work well deserving our pains to make a strict inquiry concerning the First Principles of Human Knowledge, to sift and examine them on all sides, especially since there may be some grounds to suspect that those lets and difficulties, which stay and embarrass the mind in its search after truth, do not spring from any darkness and intricacy in the objects, or natural defect in the understanding, so much as from false Principles which have been insisted on, and might have been avoided.

GEORGE BERKELEY
A TREATISE CONCERNING THE PRINCIPLES OF HUMAN KNOWLEDGE

Ultimately, a cure for Alzheimer's disease will emerge from the concerted efforts of academic research and the translation of this research to the bedside through the pharmaceutical industry. Although the industry faces an image problem now in the court of public opinion, what is known colloquially as Big Pharma has been an effective model in developing many treatments for previously intractable and quite common conditions, such as hypertension, high cholesterol levels, HIV, epilepsy, and migraine. This academic-industry partnership has even made some inroads into the problem of cancer. Yet against this backdrop of promise, it is clear that Alzheimer's is different. An indisputable fact remains: pharmaceutical treatment of Alzheimer's disease is totally inadequate. While the available medications have shown some modest symptomatic benefit, they do not affect the inexorable progression of the disease.

Without a doubt, research is ultimately the answer. But neither researchers nor academic physicians have all the knowledge they need to best handle the disease *right now*. And what about community-based physicians? Their knowledge level is even lower. In the absence of a place to turn and the lack of a system in place for dealing with the disease comprehensively, patients, families, and the medical community all feel a sense of frustration. The frustration and the powerful longing for a silver-bullet solution can lead researchers to make overly optimistic predictions about the timetable for a cure. How often do we hear about "breakthroughs" in the media, only to assume that one more glimmer of hope has been extinguished when no further news surfaces? In reality, the litany of remedies reported at the moment of initial enthusiasm are no longer newsworthy when they fail to demonstrate efficacy or, in the case of supplements, do not promise a windfall of profits and hence are inadequately studied. Perhaps a look at the research pathway—what has been called "bench to bedside"—might be enlightening.

THE ACADEMY DELIVERS
THE FUNDAMENTAL BIOLOGY

In 1984, an act of Congress directed the National Institute on Aging, a division of the National Institutes of Health, to establish a number of Alzheimer's Disease Research Centers (ADRCs).[1] In these centers, teams of nationally recognized experts have created clinical and laboratory settings for the diagnosis, treatment, and research of Alzheimer's disease. The first ADRC grant was made in 1985, and there are now twenty-nine centers, all of which are intended to provide support for new research on the disease throughout the United States. Each center is funded—currently at a total of $6.5 million—for a period of five years, after which time the centers must compete for renewal. Most of the centers have had uninterrupted funding since their inception, which suggests that the agencies awarding the grant funds consider nearly every center successful. Most federally backed research is supported—and delivered to patients— through this system of ADRCs. Those who are shepherding medications from a fundamental discovery in the university to the testing of a drug in patients—and it is a circuitous path set with many unexpected traps— often use ADRCs to conduct clinical trials. All of the centers are associated with large hospitals that offer advanced technology and highly specialized treatment. Most leading clinical Alzheimer researchers in the United States are associated with one of these centers.

Because the ADRCs are usually located in highly specialized referral centers, how well they address dementia in the community is an open question. Patients with rare or complex problems tend to gravitate to large tertiary-care centers, but Alzheimer's disease is not rare and its clinical management is not complex. What is missing in the ADRC model is a community-based program. Some centers do have a strong focus on their surrounding neighborhoods, but most do not. Among those that do focus on the community are the Boston University Alzheimer's Disease Research Center, which is involved in the care of the large local African American population, and the Mount Sinai ADRC in New York, which has programs that address issues in Latino populations. Health disparities exist not only in care delivery but also in research. Often the underserved find it most difficult to participate or remain in clinical trials. Although the efficacy of these efforts is still unclear, the intention is to address some of the health disparities in less affluent communities.

While the dissemination of health information to the community is important, we need to improve the retention rates of subjects in the scientific trials from which we draw conclusions. One recent examination of this problem of attrition reported that upward of 40 percent of participants dropped out of a two-year prospective study in France. Researchers at the University of Toulouse knew that when patients drop out of long-term studies designed to look at a group of people over time, the validity of the study results is threatened. So Nicola Coley and her colleagues set out to identify the factors that could predict whether patients with Alzheimer's disease were likely to drop out of a study. Elderly patients with cognitive impairment or Alzheimer's disease may face hurdles such as the refusal of a caregiver to participate or the loss of autonomy. Some may die during the study. Coley, an epidemiologist, studied 686 patients between the years 2000 and 2002. Although they had been diagnosed with Alzheimer's disease, many still had only mild cognitive impairment, and more than half were still independent. Of those patients, 278—or 40 percent—had dropped out at the two-year follow-up. Caregivers were a significant factor in attrition, the researchers found: "Caregiver status combined with living arrangements, and level of caregiver burden were also associated with higher attrition rates." The bottom line, they said, was that attrition can threaten the scientific validity of long-term studies that are useful—indeed, necessary—to improve our understanding of Alzheimer's disease.[2]

Equally clear is that study designs, just like Alzheimer care in general, must alleviate some of the caregiver burden to be successful.

Overall, ADRC-affiliated scientists have contributed a great deal to our fundamental understanding of Alzheimer's disease. However, the ADRC track record as an effective conduit to the community of information, care, and prevention has been more problematic.

BIG PHARMA SETS THE AGENDA

Because treatments for Alzheimer's disease have the potential to capture multibillion-dollar markets, nearly every major pharmaceutical company has an Alzheimer program. Their goals are generally the same: they hold onto one or two of the most popular ideas about the cause of the disease and, with these assumptions, chase the same culprits as the other companies. These disease culprits are the very molecules in our bodies that contribute to the cause of the disease. However, like in any crime scene, identifying the bad guy is not always easy among a group of bystander molecules whose only guilt is that of association. Identifying precisely those molecules in our bodies that lead to disease is a very challenging task. In the slang of the industry, the disease-causing molecules are called *targets*. The idea is that hitting a target with a drug will knock out the disease. In the research arena, putative targets abound, but it is rare that a target is definitively proven. The proof is when a drug delivers a bull's-eye and we cure the disease. Needless to say, we have not yet hit the target in Alzheimer's disease.

Unfortunately, pharmaceutical companies tend to operate as a pack. They look over their shoulders all the time in order to be sure they are covering all the same bases as their competitors, rather than striking out on independent paths. If one company develops a drug, other companies will not be far behind in developing a similar product. Hence in nearly every drug category we have a list of "me-too" drugs that are nearly identical. In this arena the winner, which is measured in financial gain, goes to the best marketing team. A company that ignores mainstream targets risks being left behind if other companies succeed.

Every drug starts off as a chemical until it works on a disease; then we categorize that chemical as a drug. We say a target is *druggable* if we can envision a chemical that could bind to the target and destroy its disease-causing function. Remember, of course, that targets are molecules made in our own bodies; they are there for a reason and often contribute not only to the disease but also to our health. Therefore, destroying a target can also have untoward consequences. In addition, our aim at a target is not always so precise. Sometimes we hit unintended molecules and the drug causes intolerable side effects. Finding a good drug for any disease is a minefield, and the vast majority of chemicals that initially look promising ultimately fail.

The type of drug the Alzheimer research community seeks is called a *disease-modifying drug*. This kind of drug is expected to alter the inexorable progression of a disease, in this case, the plaques and tangles in the brain and the progression of the dementia. Currently, the drugs approved by the Food and Drug Administration (FDA) for Alzheimer's disease fall into two categories. In one category are drugs called *anti-cholinesterases*, which prevent the breakdown of acetylcholine, a brain chemical believed to be important for memory and thinking. These drugs are Exelon (rivastigmine), Aricept (donepezil), and Razadyne (galantamine, now available as a generic drug). As the disease progresses, those brain cells, which make acetylcholine, die and the efficacy of these drugs wears off. In the second category is the single drug Namenda (memantine), which is an N-methyl D-aspartate (NMDA) antagonist, and is believed to work by regulating glutamate. Alzheimer patients often take Namenda in conjunction with an anticholinesterase.

Despite the laudable goal of disease modification, these few Alzheimer drugs that have modest effects on symptoms have no effect on the underlying disease progression. In effect, they are mere bandages. An analogy is taking aspirin for fever. An aspirin will lower a fever, but it will not treat the underlying cause of the fever, for example, pneumonia. That requires antibiotics. Existing Alzheimer drugs are like aspirin for fever—but less effective: unlike aspirin, which is effective in reducing fever, their likely benefit in reducing Alzheimer symptoms is modest at best. Many patients show no benefit, and the cost in terms of dollars is high. In fairness, those patients who experience some short-lived benefit—such as restoration of the ability to put on one's shoes or go to the bathroom—prove that the drugs have some value. The question is whether the small benefit in a fraction of individuals is worth the cost. If one has to parcel limited resources among many household needs such as those of the children or the caretaker, how do we weight the modest benefit of an Alzheimer medication? Is it a disservice to a loved one to withhold these medications in deference to other pressing needs? These difficult choices are not made any easier by the aggressive marketing of pharmaceutical companies, which often create a sense of guilt and misplaced priorities regarding their products. Those families who cannot afford these drugs often feel that they are denying a loved one a great deal more than what the drugs actually deliver.

Marketing campaigns rarely give figures on how well a specific drug performs because there is no requirement to do so. FDA approval does not require that a high percentage of patients will benefit from the drug; it simply requires that a pharmaceutical company show that the drug improved the lot of enough patients to satisfy statisticians. This means it is fully expected that a large percentage of users will not benefit. It is a well-kept secret that a very large number of medications will not work and are not expected to work in many people who use them. And patients may ultimately be left with opaque information, at best, about whether they will actually benefit from a drug. In other words, doctors do not usually offer information about how likely it is that a prescribed drug may or may not be effective.

Conversely, drugs that benefit only a small number of patients—not enough to be considered statistically significant—may be removed from the marketplace by the drug companies themselves. Removing the drug leaves those few people who do benefit from the drug without treatment, and therefore, it would certainly be preferable to learn more about those who did benefit. Because people differ from one another, it is not surprising that drugs may be more or less effective in different individuals. Some medications may work in only a small number of people who happen to have a particular genetic makeup that makes them responsive to the medication. However, the small profit margin for drugs that are useful for only a few people is a disincentive to development for Big Pharma. Instead, the one-size-fits-all approach continues to drive the search for the billion-dollar drug. Thus, economic drivers lead to drugs that have very few side effects, but limited beneficial effects for large numbers of people, rather than more potent drugs that can be well tolerated by smaller numbers of people.

Big Pharma's approach is conservative and risk averse, requiring that companies constantly watch their backs. Nevertheless, the goal of these pharmaceutical giants is laudable—after all, they are searching for drugs to cure disease. But there is a fine line between the creation of drugs that will heal and the marketing of drugs that will exploit the public's desperate need for treatment and aid only a fraction of the population of sufferers.

ON TO THE FOOD AND DRUG ADMINISTRATION

Twenty-five years ago, treatment for Alzheimer's disease was not discussed. It seemed too remote, and too little was known about how to attack the disease. That has all changed. Big Pharma has concluded that Alzheimer's research has sufficiently matured to justify its investment. As drugs move through industry pipelines, the final arbiter for bringing a drug to the market in the United States is the Food and Drug Administration.

From 2000 to 2008, while basic knowledge about Alzheimer's disease was exploding and the pharmaceutical industry was investing millions in drug development, the FDA often found itself without a leader or in transition between frequently changing commissioners. Jane E. Henney, MD, a Clinton appointee, served from January 17, 1999 to January 19, 2001. For nearly two years President Bush left the post empty until he selected Mark McClellan, MD, PhD, who served from November 14, 2002, to March 26, 2004. After another lengthy interval, Lester M. Crawford, DVM, PhD, served from July 18, 2005, to September 23, 2005.[3] Andrew C. von Eschenbach, MD, became FDA commissioner in December 13, 2006, and served until President Obama chose former New York City health chief Margaret Hamburg, MD, to run the agency on March 14, 2009.

One of the most difficult tasks the FDA has is to balance its two mandates. One governing force is the lobby of patients with incurable diseases, for whom the clock is ticking. The other is the agency's solemn responsibility to approve drugs that are both safe and effective. Striking a balance between ensuring public safety and promptly approving medications is the ultimate challenge. These often conflicting interests are triangulated by the pharmaceutical industry, which wants to get drugs to market to recoup its investment in drug development, but places (or misplaces) most of its clout behind blockbuster products that are as likely to remedy erectile dysfunction or baldness as they are to make a difference in an incurable disease. Where efficacy versus safety most intensely clash is among patients with diseases that are fatal or, like Alzheimer's disease, entirely destroy one's quality of life, in a relatively short time. A patient with a life expectancy of a year is willing to take more risk in trying an unproven, possibly unsafe, drug. However, the industry thwarts compassionate use of its investigational compounds in Alzheimer's disease because the occurrence of complications in a poorly controlled study could derail the drug's approval.

According to Daniel Carpenter and his Harvard colleagues, writing in the *New England Journal of Medicine*, this balancing act has been aggravated by the Prescription Drug User Fee Act, which was passed by Congress in 1992 and revised in 1997.[4] This legislation allows pharmaceutical companies to pay a "user fee" to the FDA in exchange for a ruling on a drug application within ten months for standard reviews and six months for priority reviews. Carpenter and his colleagues studied whether the introduction of drug approval deadlines has adversely affected pharmaceutical safety. They systematically collected all "new molecular entities" reviewed by the FDA from 1950 to 2004, paying particular attention to the approval time before and after the drug user fee legislation. The researchers compared the approval times with the records of post-approval safety. To assess post-approval safety, they noted whether a drug was withdrawn from the market after approval; whether a "black box warning," which suggests potentially severe adverse side effects, was added; or whether an approved dosage of a medication was later disallowed.

The results of this study were disturbing. First, the entire pattern of the approval process appeared to change after 1992. Although approval times were spread out during the four decades before 1992, after 1992 approval times tended to cluster in a two-month period immediately before the congressionally stipulated deadline. This "just in time" approval process appears to be a harbinger of postapproval safety problems: those drugs approved just before the deadline were three times more likely to be pulled from the market than drugs approved at other times in the review cycle, twice as likely to have one or more dosage forms discontinued, and up to seven times more likely to receive a black box warning. Like any good scientists, the investigators tried to find some explanation for their data other than the worrisome conclusion that the user-fee law hastened the introduction of dangerous drugs to the marketplace, but they were unable to find one. For example, it was not the case that approvals in the immediate pre-deadline period were disproportionately high risk, were totally novel types of drugs, or were linked to urgent consumer demand. Consequently, the authors concluded that buying a faster approval time under the user-fee law had a negative impact on FDA decision making.

GETTING THE BASICS RIGHT:
THE FIRST STEP TOWARD DRUG DISCOVERY

The year 1906 was notable for Alois Alzheimer's description of a woman who died with dementia at age fifty-six, now famously ensconced in history. He presented his lecture, titled "On a Peculiar, Severe Disease Process of the Cerebral Cortex," to the Thirty-seventh Assembly of Southwest German Alienists in Tübingen. (Historically, the word *alien* connotes mental alienation or estrangement, and an *alienist* is a medical professional who deals with conditions, such as insanity, that result in alienation.) One year earlier, Albert Einstein published three of the most remarkable and influential physics papers ever in a burst of creative energy, and the year 1905 became known as *Annus Mirabilis*, a Latin term that translates to "year of miracles." And in 1906, Santiago Ramón y Cajal and Camillo Golgi won the Nobel Prize in Physiology or Medicine. These two laureates invented staining techniques that revealed for the first time the complexity of brain cells. Cajal, struck with the beauty of the brain, called the elaborate branching patterns of brain cells "butterflies of the soul." In the same year, deep inside the brain examined by Alzheimer, the butterflies were gone. Instead, the brain was filled with two structures considered the classical hallmarks of the disease: *senile plaques* and *neurofibrillary tangles*. These two structures, visible only under a microscope, contain the abnormal proteins associated with Alzheimer's disease.

Alzheimer's patient, Auguste Deter, was brought to a mental institution in Frankfurt in 1901 because her husband, Karl Deter, a railroad worker, could no longer care for her while holding his job. She became irrationally jealous that her husband was having an affair with a neighbor, she hid her possessions around the house because she suspected they were being stolen, she lost interest in personal hygiene, and sometimes she would scream during the night. When Alzheimer examined her brain under the microscope after her death he observed the abnormal ropelike clumps of protein, called *neurofibrillary tangles*, that collect inside neurons and strangle the life from the cell. He also observed another structure called the *senile plaque*, a sticky, abnormal protein believed to leak from tiny blood vessels and ooze through the spaces between brain cells and puddle in plaques that surround these brain cells. While senile plaques were observed earlier by Paul Blocq and Georges Marinesco in 1892 and again by Otto Fischer in 1907, Alzheimer was the first to connect these structures to clinical dementia. His dual interests in psychiatry, a field in which he started his career at the Stadtische Irrenstalt Mental Asylum in Frankfurt, and neuropathology prepared him for his discovery. The clinical story of Frau Deter piqued his interest. When he examined her postmortem, he staked out new territory and left his indelible mark. In the same year that Alzheimer delivered his lecture in Tübingen, Emil Kraepelin, one of the leading psychiatrists of the time, invited Alzheimer to move with him to the Royal Psychiatric Clinic in Munich. As a sort of publicist for Alzheimer and his own new clinic, Kraepelin dubbed the condition Alzheimer's *krankheit*, or disease. Ironically, while Alzheimer is given enormous credit for linking the plaques and tangles to dementia, the actual relationship of these structures to the dementia—how they actually cause dementia and eventual death—is still debated today.

From these exciting years at the opening of the twentieth century until the late 1960s, Alzheimer's disease research came to a standstill. Not until 1966, with a series of papers by Bernard Tomlinson, Martin Roth, and Gary Blessed, was the next research milestone achieved. Until the publication by this English group of neurologists and neuropathologists, Alzheimer's disease was considered a rare entity that affected people in the same age group as Auguste Deter. The disease was also called presenile dementia because it affected people in their "presenium," a time in life earlier than the expected age when senile dementia was thought to occur. Cases of dementia in those over an arbitrary age, usually set at age sixty-five, were labeled senile dementia (or senility), and the cause was widely attributed to atherosclerotic vascular disease. *Sclerotic* means "hard," and so the lay term "hardening of the arteries" was used to describe the physiological process in elders with dementia. What Roth, Tomlinson, and Blessed showed was the vast majority of those over age sixty-five with dementia had the typical plaques and tangles that are signs of Alzheimer's disease. In their study they compared the brains of fifty demented elderly people to a control set. Under the microscope, half of the brains from demented individuals had clear-cut Alzheimer's disease, which came to be called *senile dementia of the Alzheimer type* (SDAT), to distinguish it from the apparently identical disease that affected people a decade or more younger. Among the remaining group with dementia, nearly a quarter had both Alzheimer's disease and atherosclerosis of brain blood vessels and had experienced multiple strokes.

At the same time, physicians who studied stroke were beginning to reach the same conclusion based on astute clinical observations. C. Miller Fisher, the leading stroke neurologist of the time, who was worshipped by his trainees at Massachusetts General Hospital, pointed out that the small strokes, called *lacunes*, were overrated as a cause of dementia. In his study of 114 consecutive patients with lacunes at autopsy, dementia was rare. Fisher noted that "lacunes lick the psyche and bite the soma, just opposite to senile dementia."[5]

These findings rekindled interest in the Alzheimer's disease. The work of Tomlinson, Roth, and Blessed brought to the fore the staggering numbers of elders likely to be affected by the disease, no longer considered rare. What had been artificially partitioned into presenile dementia and senile dementia could now be viewed as a single disease entity. It remains remarkable how long it took to discern the simple insight of the English neurological group. The technology was certainly in place to make the discovery throughout the entire period since Alzheimer's first case. By some accounts, this scientific failure was due to the societal view in Germany that elders were an expendable element of society; because of this, no one cared even to look systematically at their postmortem brains when they died of dementia.

After the publications of Roth, Tomlinson, and Blessed, the pendulum swung rapidly toward a widespread belief that Alzheimer's disease was the factor that accounts for nearly all dementia in elders. The disease was considered—and, with some modifications, still is—so common that people began to ask: Is Alzheimer's disease really a disease, or is it a consequence of normal aging—like wrinkling of the skin or cataracts or enlarged prostate in men? Based on the finding that some people reach the upper boundary of life expectancy with neither plaques nor tangles to be found in their brain tissue, most researchers concluded that Alzheimer's is a disease to which elders are particularly, but not inevitably, vulnerable. Striking examples of those who beat the odds by continuing with their creative output in their ninth decade are artist Pablo Picasso and cellist Pablo Casals. And in late 2008, Elliott Cook Carter Jr., one of America's most significant composers, walked onto the stage of Carnegie Hall at his one-hundredth birthday celebration, where the musicians played his new piece, a concerto for piano and orchestra called "Interventions."

Perhaps the most striking evidence that aging and Alzheimer's are not necessarily joined is the autopsy report on the world's oldest woman in 2008. At 115 years old and thought to be the oldest woman in the world at the time, she was mentally alert throughout her life, assertive, and full of interest in national and international politics and sports. Her normal cognition was documented by neuropsychological testing at ages 112 and 113. Remarkably, she had no plaques and vanishingly few tangles in her brain. She also had a near complete absence of atherosclerosis anywhere in her body. This case calls into question the common assumption that Alzheimer's disease or other forms of dementia will inevitably develop in any individual who lives long enough. Dr. Gert Holstege of University Medical Centre Groningen in the Netherlands, who led the study, was quoted as saying, "Our observations suggest that, in contrast to general belief, the limits of human cognitive function may extend far beyond the range that is currently enjoyed by most individuals, and that improvements in preventing brain disorders of aging may yield substantial long-term benefits." [6]

ALZHEIMER'S DISEASE RESEARCH GOES MOLECULAR

After the recognition that Alzheimer's disease is common, research picked up steam. The disease gradually revealed itself by an intense focus on the senile plaques and the neurofibrillary tangles. The central question posed in the field was: What exactly was this stuff that had been observed for so many decades under the microscope? What was the molecular composition of these diagnostic structures? The key person in getting to the bottom of the senile plaque was George Glenner, who was born in Brooklyn, graduated from Johns Hopkins University with a medical degree in 1954, and studied surgery and pathology at Mount Sinai Hospital in New York and the Mallory Institute at Boston City Hospital. From 1968 to 1980 he worked at the National Institutes of Health in Bethesda, Maryland, as chief of the section of molecular pathology before moving to the University of California at San Diego as a research pathologist and an attending physician at the medical school.

Glenner made a bold assumption—roundly criticized by scientists at the time—that led to the discovery of the protein that forms the senile plaque. The plaques are referred to as *amyloid plaques* because when they are stained so they can be viewed under the microscope, they appear similar to starch, which is what *amyloid* means. Glenner took advantage of a widely recognized observation that blood vessels in the brain, particularly those vessels on the surface of the brain called *meningeal vessels*, contained a similarly stained substance in their walls. Most people thought the material in blood vessel amyloid was different than the senile plaque amyloid, believing the similar staining pattern was simply because a starchy appearance is not very specific. More important, most people were also not terribly interested in the vascular amyloid because unlike senile plaques, it was not linked to Alzheimer's disease. But running against the tide of scientific opinion, Glenner was able to purify the vascular amyloid by peeling back the surface brain vessels—something that could not be done with the senile plaques in the substance of the brain—and immersing them in a chemical that separated the amyloid. Once he had a fairly pure substance, he loaded it on a machine that determines the exact order of each amino acid in the amyloid peptide. The instrument used by Glenner takes the peptide, which is a small protein, apart, one amino acid at a time. With this technique he revealed which amino acid, among the twenty different amino acids present in humans, is present at each position along the length of the amyloid peptide. For the first time we learned in detail the exact composition of the amyloid. In 1984 Glenner published this novel sequence of amino acids to not much more than a yawn from the scientific community. He also linked the amyloid to the plaques that occur in Down syndrome, which are now known to be identical to those in Alzheimer's disease. Not much later, the proof was in hand that the material Glenner found in the blood vessels was the same as that in the senile plaques. Thus, Glenner's discovery not only revealed the composition of the amyloid but also laid the basis for uniting all the places and conditions in which amyloid plaque was observed in the brain into a single biochemical entity.

One reason for the initial disinterest was that science was not yet ready to capitalize on this finding. Glenner's finding would sit idle in the scientific literature for nearly three years, which in the fast-moving field of molecular biology is an eternity. To build on this tiny toehold—those few amino acids reported by Glenner—science needed the vast resources of molecular biology. With the amino acids in hand, scientists next needed to find the gene that encodes those amino acids. Finding this gene became the next big quest, and many scientists wanted to claim the prize of its discovery because the gene itself would likely bring us closer to the underlying mystery of Alzheimer's disease. The fundamental dogma of biology tells us that the gene, made up of DNA, is transcribed into RNA, and the RNA is then translated into a protein. In this case, we knew the sequence of a piece of a protein and needed to work backward toward the gene. Today, making this link would take less than one minute. It is simply a computer search through the human genome database. However, in the 1980s we did not know the entire human genome, and cloning genes one by one was a long and tedious process.

Nevertheless, every biologist knew that gene cloning was essential for scientific progress. As these discoveries were being made, gene cloning moved from an esoteric procedure available only in a few labs with homemade reagents to a procedure easily performed in any reasonably well-equipped lab. Previously difficult multistep techniques were packaged into gene-cloning kits that lab technicians could use by simply adding an enzyme from tube A to some buffer material from tube B and some nucleotides from tube C to get results. All of this became codified in "Molecular Cloning: A Laboratory Manual" known casually as Maniatis after its author, Tom Maniatis, a very distinguished molecular biologist at Harvard and now at Columbia. Every molecular biology lab had a dogeared, coffee-stained spiral-bound Maniatis manual that made doing molecular biology as easy as preparing a gourmet meal.

The race from the Glenner peptide to cloning the gene that encodes amyloid heated up, and, as often happens in science, several groups discovered the gene at about the same time. However, if one must give credit to a single individual who passed the finish line moments before the others, that individual is Dmitri Goldgaber. In the fall of 1986, at the National Institutes of Health in the laboratory of the Nobel laureate Carleton Gajdusek, Goldgaber worked around the clock for weeks to get the gene. Once successful, Goldgaber did something very risky for a scientist in possession of "hot" data: he went to the Society for Neuroscience meeting in Washington, DC; showed up at a scientific session, disheveled and bleary-eyed; and requested that the moderator, John Morrison, allow him to present his data even though he was not on the program and had not submitted an abstract. He was granted permission, but only after all the other speakers had completed their presentations and the session was officially ended. Meanwhile, Goldgaber waited outside in the hall, clutching his folders of original data, a hodge-podge of blots from which he had deduced the gene.

Word had spread through the crowd that someone had cloned what came to be called the *amyloid precursor gene*, and instead of the usual drifting away from the session toward the end of the afternoon, the crowd swelled. Once Goldgaber mounted the stage and showed his transparencies (these were, after all, pre–Power Point days), it was clear he had the gene—and that he had one additional surprise. The gene was located on chromosome 21, the same chromosome that is triplicated in Down syndrome, and so Goldgaber had also explained why individuals with Down syndrome get senile amyloid plaques in their brains: with an extra copy of every gene on chromosome 21 they make more of the proteins encoded by those genes, including the product of the *amyloid precursor gene*, which leads to the senile plaques. A few months after this presentation, in early 1987, Goldgaber and two other groups published the cloning of the gene that encodes the amyloid and thus opened the modern molecular era of Alzheimer's research.

And in another one of those extraordinary ironies, seven years later, in 1995 George Glenner, who had pointed the way to the opening of the molecular era in Alzheimer's disease research, died at age sixty-seven—of a disease caused by the very amyloid he had discovered. He had contracted a rare form of an amyloid disease—not Alzheimer's disease, but rather a disease called *systemic senile amyloidosis*, in which the amyloid material fills the heart muscle and blocks its blood vessels.

What did we learn with the amyloid precursor gene in hand? Why was this advance so important? Recall that Glenner began with a piece of protein from the deposited amyloid from a brain vessel, and now we had a gene that encodes that protein, in effect telling it what to do. That is, the gene provides the instructions not only for the making the protein but also for how much to make and where in the body to make it. The next surprise was that the encoded protein was much longer than the small piece of protein Glenner had found; instead, the small piece of amyloid peptide fit inside the longer parent protein and had to be cut on its two ends to make the amyloid found in the plaques. Imagine the parent protein as a stick and a small piece of the stick somewhere along its length is excised as Alzheimer amyloid. The amino acids in proteins are held together by rather strong bonds, and the only way to cut out the small amyloid peptide from the larger parent protein is to use an enzyme. The discovery of the gene told us that there had to be two enzymes that cut the amyloid peptide out from the parent amyloid precursor protein. And so the next race was on to discover these enzymes. The enzymes were viewed as critical for discovering a treatment, because if we knew the identity of these enzymes we might be able to design drugs that could inhibit them—and thereby cure Alzheimer's. So the field charged into a search for the missing enzymes.

While brain tissue samples were being put in homogenizers and centrifuges for biochemical analyses in many labs—all part of a mission to hunt down the missing enzymes—another group of scientists with entirely different backgrounds and training were out doing fieldwork on a rare inherited form of Alzheimer's disease, the early onset form that affects the Colombian families described in chapter 1. These field workers were geneticists, and they scoured the world for these rare families with familial Alzheimer's disease in the hope that they would reveal more secrets about the genes that cause the disease. Gene-hunting techniques improved, and with enough family members affected by the disease over several generations, it was possible to find the one erroneous nucleotide out of three billion nucleotides in the genome. Gene hunters searched for mutations among remote populations the same way explorers searched centuries earlier for gems, gold, and other resources. In addition to the group of people with familial Alzheimer's disease in Colombia (discussed in chapter 1), others also turned up. The family that unlocked the next surprise was located in Calabria, at the southern tip of Italy.

The gene and the gene mutation causing Alzheimer's disease in the Calabrian family was discovered by Peter St. George-Hyslop at the University of Toronto. He named the gene presenilin. Shortly after this discovery, another geneticist, Alison Goate at Washington University in St. Louis, used the Colombian families and other families to show that mutations in presenilin are responsible for most of the cases of familial Alzheimer's disease. Now the field had two genes—the amyloid precursor gene and presenilin. But how might they be related? The answer is one of the most remarkable convergences known in science. It turns out that presenilin belongs to a larger protein complex that functions as one of the two hunted enzymes. The presenilin complex cuts the amyloid parent protein to generate one end of the deadly amyloid peptide. Thus geneticists collecting blood samples in remote villages around the world were suddenly linked to biochemists in the lab who were grinding up brain tissue to extract amyloid. The geneticists traveled great geographic distances and discovered the presenilin complex, an enzyme whose underlying substrate, the amyloid precursor protein, was being studied right next door in the labs of their colleagues.

Further bolstering the story was the discovery of mutations in the amyloid precursor gene that also led to early onset Alzheimer's disease. Although these mutations were even rarer than presenilin mutations, they did show that an error in the amyloid precursor gene alone was sufficient to cause the disease. What emerged was called the *amyloid hypothesis*, and it was intended to serve as the underlying root basis for Alzheimer's disease and the foundation upon which a cure would be built.

All but ignored, the neurofibrillary tangle sat on the sidelines. Quietly and without much fanfare the protein that forms the tangle was identified. Our group and several others shared in this discovery, but it was Yasuo Ihara at the University of Tokyo who definitively identified the tangle protein. The protein in the tangle is called tau. It is a normal protein that, for reasons that remain unclear, becomes prone to bunching up into long, ropelike structures that ultimately strangle the life from the neuron. Tau mutations were also discovered that lead not to Alzheimer's disease, but to another form of dementia called *frontotemporal dementia*. To this day we know much less about the tau limb of the disease. In addition to the amyloid in the senile plaques and tau in the neurofibrillary tangle, the Alzheimer brain loses neurons and connecting synapses, and has diminished blood flow. However, the vast majority of the effort and funding has gone to amyloid research, and much less attention has been directed toward other plausible explanations for Alzheimer's disease.

THE PLAQUE AND TANGLE CARTELS:
HOW RESEARCH WAS STYMIED

The goal of Alzheimer's research is to find a cure. While this common goal might seem to unite researchers, in fact the community can be quite fractious in its debate over the best path to a cure. Finding a cure requires some notion of what causes the disease, and that is where intense disagreement often erupts. While the amyloid hypothesis was riding high, a good scientist is trained to be a skeptic—and some pieces did not fit. For example, amyloid deposits were frequently seen in the brains of nondemented people who died of other causes. I recall a case from the MIT clinical trials unit many years ago where a woman with Alzheimer's disease came for an experimental treatment. Her husband served as the control. Both of them had extensive neuropsychological testing, which showed that she suffered from moderate dementia and he was cognitively normal. Sadly, a few weeks into the trial he was killed in a motor vehicle accident, and at autopsy his brain was found to be filled with senile plaques sufficient to meet the criteria for Alzheimer's disease. But in cases like this one, what is missing are the numerous neurofibrillary tangles that are also observed in the disease.

Another source of doubt was the observation that mice born from embryos into which the mutant amyloid precursor gene has been inserted develop amyloid plaques when they grow up, yet they have only minimal memory loss and minimal loss of neurons. On the other hand, tau did not offer a complete solution either. This protein is known to accumulate not just in Alzheimer's disease, but in many conditions that affect the brain, including so-called boxer's dementia after repeated blows to the head and in football players who sustain multiple concussions. A related form of this disorder that leads to Parkinson's disease is what afflicts Muhammad Ali. People often develop strong opinions in the face of uncertainty, and so the Alzheimer field was plagued by dogma about the underlying cause of disease and vitriolic disputes fractured the field.

Science is not like the law, where a case can be judged by a preponderance of the evidence. In science, just one fact that does not fit is enough to tear down the entire hypothesis. This idea is part of what Karl Popper discussed in his philosophy of science and the distinction between verification and falsifiability.[7] No number of verifying examples definitively proves a hypothesis, but a single counterexample disproves it. Listing the pros and cons of a hypothesis is less effective than scrutinizing those few findings that make one doubt one's conclusions.

These ideas were quite thoroughly laid out by Thomas Kuhn in his 1962 book, *The Structure of Scientific Revolutions*. According to Kuhn, after an exploratory period, researchers collectively settle upon the most accepted explanation, or what is termed a *paradigm*, and then they refine it and further develop its explanatory power during a period he calls "normal science."[8] In Alzheimer's research these epochs correspond to the pre-amyloid period and the amyloid hypothesis period that followed. During this period those researchers whose work failed to conform to the paradigm were not seen as refuting the paradigm, but as having made a mistake of some sort. This jump to concluding that the researcher, not the paradigm, is wrong will sound a familiar note to many researchers in the Alzheimer field who questioned the amyloid hypothesis.

Some researchers believe that the field sometimes ignored good science and cogent ideas in favor of a view that placed amyloid front and center. However, open debate lies at the heart of good science. Perhaps a more serious consequence of too strong a focus on amyloid was that the pharmaceutical industry embraced this dominant research hypothesis, and in doing so it failed to develop alternative treatment strategies. This effect on Big Pharma was felt across all drug companies because of the tendency in the industry—discussed earlier in this chapter—to focus on what other companies are doing rather than stand alone or strike out in a new direction. Standing alone is risky: researching new treatments can be more costly, and the failure rate for new therapies is high. When all companies are directed toward the same goal—for example, a remedy for amyloid—the success of one company can quickly spread to other companies. Pharmaceutical companies would rather dilute a single success and reap the financial benefits than to take the huge gambles and reach for more innovative solutions.

The dominance of the amyloid hypothesis has been a double-edged sword. On the one hand, some extraordinary scientific insights have emerged from the intensive study of the amyloid precursor gene. On the other hand, proponents have taken their scientific triumphs and turned them into an ideology that has stymied new and creative thinking. Intolerance for other scientific views is not the unique province of the amyloid camp. Proponents of the neurofibrillary pathology have been equally dogmatic, and at times the debate between these two camps has resembled a medieval session of scholastics ranting over the number of angels that can dance on the head of pin.

PURE ALZHEIMER'S DISEASE IS NOT
THE MOST COMMON FORM OF DEMENTIA

The time has come for another shift in our thinking that should dovetail well with this phase, as Kuhn would have it, of revolutionary science. Contrary to oft-quoted statistics, Alzheimer's disease is *not* the most common form of dementia. Most references suggest that upward of two-thirds of people with dementia have Alzheimer's disease, but in fact, the most common form of dementia goes by the much less appealing term *mixed dementia*. This finding was most clearly demonstrated in a study from Rush University Medical Center in Chicago. The researchers, writing in the journal *Neurology* in 2007, recruited eleven hundred elders from about forty retirement communities, senior housing buildings, and churches across northeastern Illinois. These people, who did not have any known dementia, gave doctors their permission to examine their brains in an autopsy after their death. Of the group, 80 percent of them had an autopsy diagnosis of dementia.[9] An earlier, smaller study reached a similar conclusion in the United Kingdom. These patients, who represent the majority of people with dementia, have more than one type of brain condition that led to their dementia.

The mix of physical causes includes both the plaques and tangles of Alzheimer's disease as well as disease of brain blood vessels affecting their ability to provide brain tissue with adequate amounts of oxygen. In patients with dementia, sometimes there is evidence of multiple small strokes. The strokes show that small amounts of brain tissue have died in various areas of the brain, but many people with small strokes are cognitively normal, so the strokes themselves may not be responsible for the dementia. Researchers offer a vague rebuttal to this problem. They say that as the small strokes add up, they reach a threshold that results in clinical dementia. Strokes in strategic brain locations contribute more than others to the ultimate appearance of dementia.

Disease found in brain blood vessels can impair blood flow even in the absence of strokes. The blood vessels involved are those of the smallest caliber, the arterioles and the tiny capillaries, so small that blood cells pass through one at a time. Capillaries are where blood ends its long journey from the heart and gives up its nutrients to the surrounding tissue. From the capillaries it begins the return, first to the lungs to obtain more oxygen and then on to the heart to get pumped again through the entire body. Exactly how the brain's blood vessels fail in dementia cases remains unclear, although there is an abundance of possible explanations. The most likely explanation is that blood vessel disease in dementia is related to blood vessel disease observed in other conditions related to aging, such as hypertension, arteriosclerosis, diabetes, obesity, chronic inflammation, and metabolic syndrome.

The relationship between tiny brain blood vessels and neurons is very complex. When neurons fire, they utilize more oxygen, triggering an increase in local blood flow to replace the oxygen used. Neurons gobble up oxygen more voraciously than any cell in the body. These changes in the immediate region of the neuron are the basis of functional brain imaging that allows us to observe those parts of the brain that are working when we are engaged in a specific task, like looking at a red rectangle or a threatening face, smelling the rich aroma of coffee, or listening to a specific piece of music. While diminished blood flow is common in Alzheimer's disease, another contributor may be the failure of impaired neurons to activate the increased blood flow of small vessels.

The bottom line is always the same: Can our ideas about the disease lead to a treatment? The very strong evidence (which will be discussed in chapter 6) that cardiovascular treatments have an effect on Alzheimer's disease suggests that vascular disease contributes to the incidence of Alzheimer's. The erroneous notion that pure Alzheimer's disease is what most commonly causes dementia is hindering progress. The recent failure of several amyloid-based drugs may be the result of employing a therapy that overlooks the impact of potentially diseased brain blood vessels. We might even be able to clear the brain of the dreaded plaques that are viewed as the culprit in Alzheimer's, but without attention to the blood vessels the patient will not see any clinical improvement. Drugs that may be effective in pure Alzheimer's disease may be less so when applied to those patients in whom mixed dementia is so prevalent. In some cases patients in clinical trials who are believed to have pure Alzheimer's disease may actually have mixed dementia, and therefore they may not respond to an otherwise perfectly good Alzheimer drug. One might envision that a treatment for Alzheimer's disease will require a cocktail of drugs that targets the amyloid plaques, the neurofibrillary tangles, and the blood vessels.

NEW DIRECTIONS

As this epoch of normal science in Alzheimer's research comes to a close, as contrary findings become more numerous and more troubling, we are entering the period Kuhn called revolutionary science. We are leaving a period when thinking about amyloid dominated the field and entering a post-amyloid era that integrates the insights about amyloid with novel ways to think about biology. What is emerging from this new tack is no longer based on what we see under the microscope—the senile plaques and the neurofibrillary tangles. The new research is based on a much less obvious biology built from large data sets capable of detecting a change in nearly every gene without any bias or preconception that one's favorite gene—whether the amyloid precursor gene or *tau* gene—is the culprit.

The roots of current promising research lie in what we call *systems biology*, a term that struck reverence in the heart of biologists when it was first introduced but has rapidly became so encompassing and diluted that its meaning has become passé just as its approach has become pervasive. The idea behind systems biology was to wean us from focusing only on a single favorite gene—for example, the amyloid precursor gene—and instead view the organism as an entire system. The implications carried a profound shift in thinking because biologists, like many scientists, often pride themselves on being reductionists. They believe that a complete knowledge of every gene individually will eventually lead to knowledge of the entire organism. But this is not true. Instead, a wealth of data has appeared over the past decade that describes systems properties of organisms that could not be predicted from knowing each individual component. In other words, we are not a simple sum of all our individual genes, but a complex network of these genes that includes their many interactions and relationships. Researchers came to recognize that no matter how much we learn about a single gene, we still need to know how a gene integrates itself into the overall function of an organism. Even a so-called lethal gene can be benign when its effects are mitigated by the setting in which it operates. Aging is a quintessential systems problem; no single gene controls it.

Diseases that may be classified very differently often turn out to have surprising connections when viewed from a systems perspective. The *diseasome*, a term coined by Albert-Laszlo Barabasi, a physicist at Northwestern University,[10] attempts to get at these connections. For example, Niemann-Pick disease type C is a fatal inherited disorder in which lipids accumulate to harmful levels in the spleen, liver, lungs, bone marrow, and brain of children. The cause is a mutation in a gene involved in lipid metabolism. So it is totally surprising that like Alzheimer's disease, Niemann-Pick has neurofibrillary tangles. Connections such as these will open new therapeutic opportunities because drugs now used for one disease might be effective in related conditions.

Because Alzheimer's disease is so inextricably tied to aging, one cannot completely disentangle it. Thus we have traveled full circle from the transformative views of major researchers such as Roth, Tomlinson, and Blessed, who taught us that Alzheimer's disease is not simply the inevitable consequence of aging, but is a disease to which elders are particularly vulnerable. Perhaps we might see our progress as a spiral rather than a circle because we are returning to the link between aging and dementia, but with a fresh view that the aging process itself is tractable, that the specific components of aging that contribute to Alzheimer's disease can be dissected and perhaps remedied. Using different model organisms from yeast to the tiny worm *C. elegans* to fruit flies to laboratory mice, we can now increase longevity and in the process ward off age-related conditions.

Prominent among the ravages of aging is a condition called *metabolic syndrome*, which represents the combination of hypertension, poor control of blood sugar levels leading to diabetes, elevated "bad" cholesterol, elevated triglycerides, and obesity. The condition may affect as many as 25 percent of the US population and is a significant risk for the development of Alzheimer's disease for those who survive into their sixties or seventies. A recent study from Brazil by Matheus Roriz-Cruz found that in a group of people over age sixty, those with metabolic syndrome had lower scores in every category of brain function, including cognition, planning, neuromotor skills, functional abilities, and depression. The differences between those with and those without metabolic syndrome increased with age.[11]

Cynthia Kenyon, a molecular biologist at the University of California at San Francisco, has touted *C. elegans* as a model for aging.[12] She has observed these tiny worms entering their dotage and claims that their pockmarked appearance when viewed under a microscope is the result of the progressive loss of cells, a condition that resembles metabolic syndrome. Many scientists have observed that restricting calories in the worm can prevent this syndrome and significantly extend their lives.[13] The finding that caloric restriction extends life span has now been replicated in many different species, including nonhuman primates.

Once scientists could observe a trait in worms, they were on their way to finding those genes that control the trait. (We refer to traits such as life span, height, or hair color as *phenotypes*.) Indeed, it was not long before a gene family called the *sirtuins* was found that contributed to the regulation of life span. Interestingly, members of this gene family are found in organisms as diverse as yeast and humans, and in all these organisms the gene is likely to have an effect on life span.

Sirtuins are enzymes—proteins produced by cells to speed up a chemical reaction and sirtuins are likely to speed up reactions that can slow the aging process. In the view of pharmacologists, sirtuins are "druggable targets." This term refers to the selection of one molecule in the human body from among its millions of constituents based on identifying its function that can be harnessed to ameliorate some condition. Sirtuins fit the bill—they appear to have a function in slowing aging and we can potentially boost their function with a drug. To find that drug, the chemist studies the chemical structure of the biomolecule in the hope of finding a drug that can bind to the biomolecule and, in the case of the sirtuins, push its function into high gear. In what might be called a systems approach, David Sinclair of the Harvard Medical School and his colleagues at a company called BIOMOL screened many compounds in their search for those with some effect on the enzyme activity of sirtuins.[14]

Their screen blindly probed the atomic space surrounding the enzyme by mixing one compound after another with the enzyme until they found one that had the activity they sought. It is a tedious process that is only possible to do with robots because of the hundreds of thousands of compounds screened. Success is based on the sheer numbers of compounds screened, the savvy with which those compounds are selected, and a good dose of luck. Remarkably, what emerged from this screen in 2003 was the compound resveratrol, which is found in the skin of red grapes and is present in red wine. Resveratrol increases sirtuin activity. However, the amounts of resveratrol in red wine are not large enough to do the job. The beneficial effects needed could not be obtained from a daily glass, nor even a bottle, of red wine. One way that we know how much resveratrol is needed is from a mouse study published by Sinclair in 2006.[15] The presence of resveratrol changed the physical makeup of middle-aged mice on a high-calorie diet to that of mice on a standard healthy diet and significantly increased their survival.

Again using systems biology approaches, the investigators simultaneously tracked thousands of genes to find those that changed on a high-calorie diet. They found that of the 153 genes that changed their expression when the mice were on a high-calorie diet, 144 underwent changes when resveratrol was introduced. To date, the only human experimental trial conducted used extremely high doses of resveratrol—three to five grams—in a proprietary formulation owned by the biotech company Sirtris Pharmaceuticals in Cambridge, Massachusetts, to lower blood sugar. Definitive results and follow-up trials have not yet been reported.

Another enzyme now getting deserved attention is histone deacetylase, which the body uses to shut off certain sets of genes at precisely the right time. Inhibiting the histone deacetylase has the opposite effect; it turns genes on. Many researchers are developing selective inhibitors of this enzyme family, which have the potential to restore function to the brain even after it has undergone some degeneration. In a remarkable study by Li-Huei Tsai, director of the Picower Institute at MIT and a member of the Scientific Advisory Board of Sirtris, inhibiting this enzyme family was actually able to restore memories that were lost during the neurodegenerative process.[16]

Tsai put a gene into a mouse that causes the brain to degenerate. Placing genes in mice has become standard technology—the cloned gene is injected into the fertilized egg cell of a mouse, the gene integrates into the mouse DNA, and as the mouse develops it carries the injected gene, known as a *transgene*. In this case, Tsai constructed the transgene in such a way that she could turn it on and off at will simply by feeding the mouse an antibiotic. Before she turned the gene on, she taught the mouse how to find some food in a maze. Then she turned the gene on, and as the mouse's brain began to degenerate it forgot where the food was located in the maze. She then treated the mouse with an inhibitor of histone deacetylase—and, surprisingly, the mouse recovered its memory of where the food was located in the maze. The study raises profound questions about the potential for retrieval of memories we may have considered irretrievably lost. Although the compound she used in the mice cannot be used in humans because of its toxicity, the study opens the way to another category of proteins that might be targeted by drugs of the future. The search for highly specific, nontoxic histone deacetylase inhibitors is under way.

Another promising direction is prompting the cell's waste disposal system to do a better job of removing damaged proteins that accumulate in neurons. Cells have a complex system for recognizing damaged proteins, attempting to repair them, and, if the repair fails, discarding them. Failure to correct or discard a damaged protein can lead to impairment of the entire cell. Proteins used for repair are called *chaperones* or *heat shock proteins*. Two proteins that interact must fold correctly to fit together, and these proteins help other proteins to fold into a shape necessary to do their job. The term *heat shock* points to the tendency for proteins to misfold when the temperature changes even a small amount—remember, the body expends a lot of energy to maintain our temperatures within a narrow range, slightly above or below 98.6 degrees Fahrenheit. These tight temperature boundaries give nature more latitude in utilizing proteins because temperature resistance does not have to be built into their structures. If a protein becomes damaged, heat shock proteins attach to the damaged protein and help to restore its function. The tau protein in the Alzheimer neurofibrillary tangle is an example of a misfolded damaged protein that gums up the cell because it has not been appropriately removed by the cell's waste disposal system.

Although no drugs have been developed yet that target misfolded tau protein, the cancer field has also been interested in protein misfolding because a similar problem affects other proteins in cancerous cells. Drugs are under investigation for cancer treatment that target one of these chaperone proteins called *heat shock protein 90*. One class of these drugs moving through the pharmaceutical pipeline was developed by Gabriela Chiosis at the Memorial Sloan-Kettering Cancer Institute,[17] and these compounds certainly deserve testing in Alzheimer's disease. Other scientists have explored a link between Alzheimer's disease and diabetes. These links are based on the following evidence: an epidemiological association in which having diabetes increases one's risk for Alzheimer's disease, Alzheimer patients may have insulin dysfunction in their brains, certain enzymes operate in pathways related to both diseases, and preliminary data that the drug might boost mental function in some Alzheimer patients. The pharmaceutical giant Glaxo Smith Kline believed the link was sufficiently strong that it launched a multimillion-dollar study of the diabetes drug Avandia (rosiglitazone). Unfortunately, this drug failed in an Alzheimer's disease trial, but the underlying thinking behind the trial may still have merit.

Extending the indications of existing drugs—especially drugs that are already approved—to new diseases is a powerful strategy for the industry. In these cases all the work involved in safety, dosing, and formulation have been completed. The company need only demonstrate efficacy, and it is ready to file with the FDA. For example, the drug valproic acid, first used to treat seizures, has had its use extended and is now approved to treat mood disorders, particularly the manic phase of bipolar disorder, and migraine. Even before filing for a use beyond what the drug was originally approved for, physicians are allowed to prescribe it for other conditions, and therefore sales start to rise before FDA approval for the new indication is secured. However, pharmaceutical companies are not allowed to market the drug for these off-label uses until the drug is officially approved.

Stem cells offer another therapy on the more distant horizon. The use of stem cells as a repair tool for the damage inflicted by Alzheimer's disease remains difficult to envision because the damage is so extensive. But as a remedy for more specific neurodegenerative conditions like Parkinson's disease, in which cell death is limited to a specific part of the brain, stem cells do indeed offer hope.

Embryonic stem cells have the potential to become any cell in the body while at the same time retaining their identity as a stem cell. How do they manage this unique trick? What defines a stem cell is its unique way of dividing. Usually, when cells divide the two daughter cells are nearly equivalent. When stem cells divide they parcel their contents asymmetrically to the daughter cells. One daughter cell differentiates into a specific cell type, such as a neuron, and the other daughter cell remains a stem cell that retains the ability to proliferate. Too much "stemness" in one daughter cell and the result could be cancer, which is the uncontrolled proliferation of cells. Too much fate determination, that is, the markings that direct its destiny, in a daughter cell and degeneration could be the outcome. Cancer and degeneration may emerge from the dual and radically divergent identities of stem cells. The seeds of the Alzheimer disease process may lie buried in the primordial stem cells that give rise to those neurons affected by the disease. Building the web of interconnections between stem cells, cancer, and aging will enlarge the scope of treatment possibilities for Alzheimer's disease.

It is well known that when cells divide, all the daughter cells inherit the same DNA from the parental cells, and stem cells are no exception. Thus, every cell in your body has the same DNA you inherited from your parents, which was originally derived from the stem cells that marked your beginning. But even though all the daughter cells derived from stem cells have the same DNA, stem cell progeny can assume many different identities—neurons, hair follicles, kidney cells, and so on. The ability to assume many different identities with the same complement of DNA is called *epigenetics*, and this concept is reshaping much of our thinking about biomedicine.

The long-term fate of stem cell offspring may lie deep within its inner workings. Long after stem cell progeny assume their final identity, perhaps as a neuron, a disease may be lying in wait. The moment at which a cell's destiny becomes Alzheimer's disease is unknown, but we do know that the rare gene mutations that cause Alzheimer's disease are present in the stem cells. Casting one's fate at the moment of conception carries a mythic echo. Like Aphrodite, life's stages are bundled into the primordial state. Aphrodite was a composite of three goddesses called Inanna, Ishtar, and Astarte: the maiden who rose every morning to renew her youthful beauty, followed by the fullness of motherhood, and then the gradual waning of her power and strength, while planting the seed of wisdom for the next cycle even as she faded into the night. These mythological stages serve as a wonderful metaphor for much of biology.

NOTES

1. For a list of all twenty-nine centers, see US National Institutes of Health, National Institute on Aging, "AD Research Centers," Alzheimer's Disease Education & Referral Center, http://www.nia.nih.gov/Alzheimers/ResearchInformation/ResearchCenters (accessed May 19, 2009).

2. Nicola Coley et al., "Predictive Factors of Attrition in a Cohort of Alzheimer Disease Patients," *Neuro-epidemiology* 31 (2008): 69–79, published online July 12, 2008, content.karger.com/produktedb/produkte.asp?typ=pdf&file=000144087 (accessed June 15, 2009).

3. Lester M. Crawford Jr., remarks at the FDA Public Meeting on Bar Code Labeling for Drugs, July 26, 2002, http://www.fda.gov/NewsEvents/Speeches/ucm054041.htm (accessed February 4, 2010).

4. D. Carpenter et al., "Drug-Review Deadlines and Safety Problems," *New England Journal of Medicine* 358 (2008): 1354–61.

5. C. M. Fisher, "Lacunes: Small, Deep Cerebral Infarcts," *Neurology* 15 (1965): 774–84. Fisher also writes on dementia in an article "Dementia in Cerebral Vascular Disease," in *Cerebral Vascular Disease*, 6th conference, ed. R. Siekert and J. Whisnant (New York: Grune and Stratton, 1968), pp. 232–36.

6. W. F. den Dunnen et al., "No Disease in the Brain of a 115-Year-Old Woman," *Neurobiology of Aging* 29, no. 8 (2008): 1127–32.

7. Karl Popper, *The Logic of Scientific Discovery* (London: Routledge, 2002), p. 18.

8. Thomas Kuhn, *The Structure of Scientific Revolutions*, 3rd ed. (Chicago: University of Chicago Press, 1996), p. 10.

9. J. Schneider et al., "Mixed Brain Pathologies Account for Most Dementia Cases in Community-Dwelling Older Persons," *Neurology* 69 (2007): 2197–2204, published online June 13, 2007, http://www.neurology.org/cgi/content/abstract/69/24/2197 (accessed June 25, 2009).

10. "Network Medicine—From Obesity to the 'Diseasome,'" *New England Journal of Medicine* 357 (2007): 404–407.

11. M. Roriz-Cruz et al., "Metabolic Syndrome, Successful and Pathological Neuroaging in a Stroke-Free Elderly Population," *Alzheimer's and Dementia* 4, no. 4 (2008): T706–T707.

12. Cynthia Kenyon, "*Ponce d'elegans*: Genetic Quest for the Fountain of Youth," *Cell* 84, no. 4 (1996): 501–504.

13. Malene Hansen et al., "A Role for Autophagy in the Extension of Lifespan by Dietary Restriction in *Caenorhabditis elegans*," *PLoS Genetics* 4, no. 2 (2008): e24.

14. Jason Pontin, "An Age-Defying Quest (Red Wine Included)," *New York Times*, July 8, 2007, http://www.nytimes.com/2007/07/08/business/yourmoney/08stream.html (accessed February 4, 2010).

15. David A. Sinclair et al., "Resveratrol Improves Health and Survival of Mice on a High-Calorie Diet," *Nature* 444 (2006): 337–42.

16. D. Kim et al., "Deregulation of HDAC1 by p25/Cdk5 in Neurodegeneration," *Neuron* 60 (2008): 803–17.

17. G. Chiosis et al., "Roles of Heat-Shock Protein 90 in Maintaining and Facilitating the Neurodegenerative Phenotype in Tauopathies," *Proceedings of the National Academy of Sciences* 104, no. 22 (May 29, 2007): 9511–16, http://www.ncbi.nlm.nih.gov/pubmed/17517623?dopt=Citation.

4

THE MEDICAL MODEL
HITS THE SHOALS

Lastly, inasmuch as all men, whether barbarous or civilized, everywhere frame customs, and form some kind of civil state, we must
not, therefore, look to proofs of reason for the causes and natural
bases of dominion, but derive them from the general nature or
position of mankind.
— Baruch Spinoza, *Theologico-Political Treatise* (1670)

WHAT IS THE MEDICAL MODEL?

How do doctors decide what treatment to give to their patients? The answer, in large part, lies in something called the *medical model*. Throughout years of medical school, residency, and fellowships, doctors are drilled in the tenets of the medical model. Simply put, the medical model mandates that any medical encounter focus on disease. The problem from the outset is that whatever your issue—whatever your reason for seeing the doctor—it has to fit with something in the medical textbooks. Without this *sine qua non*, the doctor-patient interaction cannot even get off the ground. However, only a fraction of us have a disease; for the remainder of us the problem is not a disease but rather avoiding disease, or worrying about a disease, or risk for a disease.

According to the medical model, avoiding disease, prevention, healthy lifestyles, and the like fall outside the scope of the field—outside what a doctor can provide. In fact, the medical model works best if a person has only one disease because coordination among different medical specialists is plagued by poor communication. But among the elderly, very few have only a single medical condition. Furthermore, the medical model requires that the disease is readily treatable by one or the other of the only two tools in the physician's armamentarium: prescription drugs or surgery. These unspoken tendencies of the medical profession leave a huge gap between the kind of health services people want and what the doctor can actually provide. Although all of us desire good health, the medical system is interested in only a single facet of good health: that which falls within the medical model.

The medical model is highly formulaic, based on observation and the stubborn facts of physical evidence. It is imparted in every medical school and built into what physicians must include in their records to be reimbursed for their services. Any patient who has worn a flimsy paper gown in an examining room has experienced the medical model firsthand. The sequence of inquiries begins with the chief complaint: the reason the patient came to see the doctor. There is no faster way to try the patience of the doctor than to rattle off a list of chief complaints. The time allotted permits only a single chief complaint, requiring patient and doctor to either choose one complaint or give short shrift to all of them.

Once the chief complaint is identified, the next part of the exam is called the history of the present illness, which details the course and specific symptoms related to the chief complaint. The history goes on to sections called past medical history, family history, social history, and review of systems. During the review of systems, the physician ticks off each organ system—heart, lungs, gastrointestinal, urinary, and so on—and inquires about problems with each. This is the last chance for the patient who is concerned about more than one thing to squeeze in another complaint. However, too many of these add-ons and the physician will label you with the medical insider term "a positive review of systems." This insult is intended to convey that whatever the query about any ailment, the patient admits to a problem.

With the history complete, the physician gets out of the chair and proceeds to the physical examination, which, according to medical training, must assess every organ system. However, depending on the complaint, the physician may choose to emphasize certain parts of the physical exam. For cognitive issues, memory testing and other spheres of cognition are assessed in detail. Based upon the history and physical exam, the physician selects a set of tests to order from the lab, which usually involves taking a sample of one or more bodily fluids and some-times a trip to the radiology suite. However, even before the test results are in, the physician's report includes a provisional diagnosis—or, if the case is problematic, a list of possible diagnoses—and a suggested treat-ment plan.

The medical model requires that the physician do her best for the patient within the bounds of current medical teachings. If a treatment—no matter how beneficial—falls outside of the medical model, the physi-cian is unlikely to recommend it. Indeed, a doctor may not even be aware of techniques and treatments that she has not learned about in a medical school classroom or a study in a professional journal. The physician is trained to do what is best for the patient by the book, but that may not lead to the best outcome for the patient. Increasingly, nonpharmacological interventions that can improve cognition or slow cognitive decline are appearing in the literature. Whether these inter-ventions involve structured cognitive challenges, lifestyle adjustments, or dietary modifications, most physicians are not prepared to discuss these options since they fall outside the medical model—and because few resources exist for patients to learn about these approaches on their own, their needs go unmet.

But it is not only the patient who suffers from this care gap. In the long decline that occurs between the initial encounter with a doctor and the final stages of Alzheimer's, spouses and family members assume the burden of caregiving—a burden that can feel heavier with each passing month. In many cases, the spouse is frail and elderly, struggling to meet the daily needs of their loved one yet loath to let go.

For Catherine Boland, the first signs of Alzheimer's surfaced eight years ago, and they were classic: she began repeating herself and doing the same things over and over again.[1] "We had her checked out," her husband, Ronald, says now. "The doctor said it was fine. We came to our own conclusions that she may have a dementia problem." At first, her short-term memory seemed somewhat intact, and she also recalled scenes and stories about her parents from fifty years ago. Lately, how-ever, her condition has worsened.

"Now, she has trouble with both," says Ronald, an eighty-four-year-old retired production manager for an electronics plant who lives north of Boston. (Pseudonyms have been used to identify all family members.) "Not only does she not remember the past, but she doesn't remember the present, as well. We'll go to a restaurant and our waitress will come over and my wife will say, 'Oh, you're working today. It's so nice to see you.' Then when the waitress comes back, she gets very confused. She's always repeating herself. She'll say again, 'Oh, it's so nice to see you.' She doesn't remember she's already met her. Or she'll take a sip of her drink at the restaurant and a few minutes later, she'll ask, 'Is that my drink?' And I'll say, 'Yeah, that's your drink,' and she doesn't remember. Or she'll eat half of her bread roll at dinner and then later I'll ask her why doesn't she finish the rest of her bread and she'll say, 'That's not mine.'"

The family took Catherine to a psychiatrist at one point, but the medication he prescribed "completely flipped her around," Ronald says. "She became completely depressed, so we decided to take her off of it." Her latest doctor has prescribed Namenda (memantine), the first drug approved by the Food and Drug Administration to treat the symptoms of moderate to severe Alzheimer's disease, and Razadyne (galantamine hydrobromide), a cholinesterase inhibitor. Ronald says he has not noticed any side effects.

But the disease has stolen elements of Catherine's personality. A retired plant manager, she was friendly and outgoing as a younger woman. Over the past two years she has become increasingly paranoid. It especially afflicts her at night, her husband says. "She's afraid. In the nighttime, she won't go from one room to the next. Not by herself. Even in the daytime, she won't go into a room first or outside of the house first. She'll say, 'Go ahead, I'll follow you.' She doesn't remember where to put her coat. She doesn't know where forks or dishes go."

Catherine's paranoia has a striking flip side: a loving embrace of strangers. She scatters hugs and kisses wherever she travels. "We went out for Thanksgiving and she was telling everybody, 'It's always so nice to see you.' She's very, very outgoing and very friendly—to everybody." Since the disease gained a foothold, Ronald says, "She thinks she knows everybody and is friends with everybody." Catherine and Ronald's daughter Anne says the disease has stripped away the vestiges of Irish reserve in her mother. "Now she's always kissing and hugging my father at restaurants. I didn't grow up with that. I don't know who this person is," she says with a laugh, "which is really nice. Having cared for my aunt—my mother's sister—I know the extremely negative reactions people with Alzheimer's can have. My mother doesn't. She is very happy."

To help care for Catherine, Ronald has enlisted his son Bob, who has moved in with them. "The biggest challenge," Bob says, "is that [my mother] is so attached to my father. She would never go anywhere without him. He never gets a chance to find out what's out there. The help is there, but she's glued to him."

He is puzzled by the vagaries of memory. Some days, she seems aware that something is amiss. "She doesn't come out and say it, but she'll joke and say, 'I'm crazy, Bob. Am I crazy, Bob?' And I'll tell her, 'I don't know; someone around here is crazy. Maybe it's me.'" Her long-term memory sends stories from the old days to the surface every now and again. She remembers the way to the shop where Ronald used to work and can list the names of people she knew as a young woman. "She remembers everything backwards, from years ago," Bob says.

Bob and Ronald's daily routine is laden with chores. As is the case with many Alzheimer's patients, washing and showering can be an ordeal. When she showers, she screams in terror. "I was outside shoveling last week and my mother was in the shower," Bob says. "The noise in the bathroom was unbelievable. She screams and hollers in the shower, but we don't know why."

Anne also helps out by taking them out one day during the week. The daily routine is exacting; Ronald takes his wife's physical needs and psychic needs into account. "If I go through the normal day, I prepare her breakfast; I take her into the bathroom and get her clothes for her," he says. Even the simplest tasks, however, must be accompanied by painstaking instruction. "I tell her exactly what to do. I turn the water on for her and make sure it's not too hot, or she won't go in. I have to prepare everything for her. She has gotten a little moody recently because she thinks I'm just being bossy by telling her what to do, so it gets kind of hard in a way."

Anne observes that her mother was always the executive in charge of the house, cleaning and cooking and organizing. Now, she says, her father and brother do everything from making meals to dusting to laying out Catherine's clothing. "She can write, she can do things, but it's easier for my dad to take her to lunch every day. It's easier than him having to cook and clean up and everything. My mother loves going out. When she gets back, she says, 'When are we going out?'"

Catherine seems to have moments of clarity; her daughter believes that at some level, she is aware of what is happening to her. "Once in awhile she'll hear my father and me talking," Anne says, "and she'll say, 'I don't have Alzheimer's, do I?' And my father will say, 'You have some kind of memory loss.' And she laughs and then five minutes later she's not going to remember what you just said. She will say sometimes, 'I don't know what's the matter with me, I can't remember.' Or I'll ask her what she did during the day and she just came back from being out and she'll say, 'I don't know what I did. I did nothing.' Because she really doesn't remember."

Anne's visits with her mother are imbued with sweetness, and she and other relatives have crossed the divide that confronts most care-givers. They have set aside old expectations and outdated notions of who their mother is and consigned the family hierarchy they grew up with to memory. They are reconstituting a new tribe with new roles and finding strength in places they may have least expected. What is her weekly visit like? "My mother just looks at me and says, 'Oh, why are you here? Can I hold your hand?' She will interrupt you with a request for a kiss. My son commented recently that he was sitting across from my mother for dinner and he tried to find a thread to continue talking with her and he couldn't. She kept interrupting him and said [referring to Anne], 'Is that your wife? The one sitting next to you? Oh, I don't envy her.' It's so funny to listen to."

One pleasure that remains, it seems, is music, so Ronald has a stack of CDs available for her, and he plays disc jockey, picking and playing the tunes. "She never gets sick of it. She claps [to the music]. She is always clapping. Sometimes in church, I'll see her put her hands together like she wants to clap, but she won't do it loudly because we're in church."

One of Ronald's biggest struggles is with Catherine's personal hygiene. And, he reflects, it would be an issue for his wife even in full-time nursing care. "If I really needed help," he says, "it would be to help her take care of herself. She's incontinent. It's very difficult for me, and I would love to have somebody help her take care of her personal hygiene, but she wouldn't have that. If she were in a nursing home, she'd have no trouble with food or even the place, but helping her dress and that kind of thing . . . well, she won't even let me help her with that, really. If she is in the bathroom and makes a mess accidentally, she denies it. She'll say, 'That wasn't me that did that.' She gets bitter, very embarrassed about it. The housework? Bob and I take care of that. The personal hygiene is the hard part. I'd really like help with that."

Ronald and Bob have talked about getting a female caregiver to help them during the day, but Catherine wouldn't hear of it. She has wandered off, as well—a common feature of the disease that makes caregivers feel they must be hypervigilant. Ronald recalls the night he fell asleep while he and Catherine were watching television. "I woke up, and she was gone. So I got in my car and I was riding around, and I saw her at the end of the street walking back. And I said, 'Where'd you go?' And she said, 'I went to church.' And I told her that nothing was going on at church. And she said, 'I know. I found that out.'"

At other times, Ronald says, Catherine will inquire about the day's agenda. "'Are we going out? Can we go out again?' She'll have her coat on and her pocketbook and she sometimes threatens to go someplace. I take her coat off for her, and turn on some music, and she forgets about it. But it makes me nervous, that she threatens to leave. She's scared stiff, though. That's the only thing holding her back. It'll be 9 p.m. and we're ready to lock up the ship, and she'll ask me, 'Are we going out?' And then she'll look outside, and say, 'Oh, it's dark out.' And that's the end of it, thank God. Because I'm not one for driving around at night.'"

Yet he is grateful for her presence and, although his job as full-time caregiver seems daunting, he says he is never tired.

Many caregivers are reluctant to step up to a new level of assistance at home or in a program—it seems like a benchmark of permanent decline that can require a psychic adjustment. Ronald Boland has not wanted additional help at home so far, his daughter says, fearing that it will be even harder on Catherine.

"I would have thought it would be worth it to try," Anne says. "I'm guessing she wouldn't cooperate. But she wouldn't remember it five minutes later. It's not like she's going to hold it against my dad. He's never been willing to let them in, to try it. It's very difficult."

Personal care is a continued struggle because it seems to feel like an assault for Catherine, her daughter surmises. "My mother reacts terribly to getting her toenails and fingernails cut. I think she would remember doing this in the past, but I really don't know. The screaming that goes on is awful. And it doesn't matter who's there, who's around. She'll scream and scream. It takes about a half hour of convincing before she'll let me do it. Most of the time we have to say to her, 'We're not going to take you out if we can't trim your nails,' because she has these long, beautiful nails. But they get way too long. She could scratch people. She wants to shake everybody's hand."

Asked to speculate on what her father needs most, and she responds with two words: time alone. "I would love to have her go to daycare, even if it's one day a week." But her mother does not want to go any-where without her father, and "he wouldn't have it. It would be a set-ting with other people, and she thinks she knows everybody so it might be really good for her. It would give my dad a break. That was maybe five years ago that someone made the suggestion. I don't know if he's afraid, maybe, that she'll be miserable. And he doesn't want her to be miserable. But she'd never remember that she did it."

Cast against a backdrop of an all-encompassing, life-altering disease such as Alzheimer's, it is clear that medicine addresses only a narrow slice of troubles—most of them after the patient is ill. Yet the patient's life in the world—as a citizen, as a functioning member of society—

needs to be considered more fully. In fact, medicine can sometimes be a powerful weapon of social change. Many social ills lead to poor health. Studies in medical journals, and treatment protocols themselves, can have larger effects on the health of the general population. Large-scale decisions of governments that affect occupational exposures and injuries, product safety, and disaster mitigation have a significant impact on the health of a society. When medicine, politics, and social movements collide, the result can be powerful for clinicians, for patients, and for history. With no survivors to push public policy forward, the soft power of medical research—and even individual doctors—could play a primary role in focusing attention on Alzheimer's.

MEDICINE AND SOCIAL CHANGE

Over the last 150 years, leaders in medicine have left just this kind of legacy: from Rudolf Virchow, who pushed for antipoverty campaigns and increased sanitation in the mid-nineteenth century, to Anthony Fauci, who redeployed all the research in his laboratory toward fighting the new AIDS virus, to Bernard Lown, a Boston cardiologist who founded a group devoted to nuclear disarmament.

Let's start with Virchow: In 1869 the German pathologist stepped into the public square when he presented a motion for disarmament to the Prussian parliament, "noting that while funding for weapons was increasing, moneys for education had remained stagnant."[2] Trained more than a century ago, Virchow believed it was morally necessary to look beyond the clinical setting and treat underlying causes of disease, such as poverty and poor public health infrastructure.

Now considered a patron saint of the public health movement, Virchow was a mentor and an example of how medicine could influence social policy for doctors like Paul Farmer. Farmer, the doctor who caught the attention of the Obama administration after founding Partners in Health, has made it a life mission to cure life-threatening infectious diseases in the poorest countries in the world. Writing about Farmer in his book *Mountains beyond Mountains*, author Tracy Kidder notes that Virchow was the first to suggest that individual cells, with the capacity to change and reproduce, were the most basic units of the body. Breaking from the medical theories of the early nineteenth century, which held that "humors" inside the body caused disease, Virchow linked illness to cellular changes.

Virchow theorized that epidemics were the result of poor sanitation, poor nutrition, and other social conditions that governments were doing little to relieve. As a young doctor, Virchow was sent by the German government to a region known as Upper Silesia to report on an epidemic of fever. Virchow was dismissed after he reported on the harrowing lives of the impoverished peasants. As Kidder writes, "This was forty years before medical science identified all the biological sources of relapsing fever—its vector is the louse—but subsequent discoveries would show that Virchow was right. Epidemics of the illness usually occur after social upheavals, in the ensuing overcrowding, poor hygiene, and malnutrition. In his report, Virchow expressed a fundamental law of epidemiology: 'If disease is an expression of individual life under unfavorable conditions, then epidemics must be indicative of mass disturbances of mass life.' His prescription for curing Upper Silesia was 'full and unlimited democracy.'"

It is at this nexus, where the physician's training and moral sense meet social distress, that Farmer and others took inspiration. "Virchow had a comprehensive vision," Farmer told Kidder. "Pathology, social medicine, politics, anthropology. My model."[3]

Almost a century later, another physician jumped into the political fray, rallying his colleagues in the United States and in Russia to the cause of nuclear disarmament. Bernard Lown, a Boston cardiologist who became a pioneer in research on sudden cardiac death and invented the defibrillator, launched Physicians for Social Responsibility in 1962 at his home in Newton, Massachusetts.

If every social rupture begins with an epiphany, Lown's occurred in 1961, when he was an assistant professor at the Harvard School of Public Health. Another postdoctoral trainee, Roy Menninger, a Quaker, asked Lown to accompany him to a lecture in Cambridge, Massachusetts, by Philip Noel-Baker, a British academic and pacifist who won the Nobel Peace Prize in 1959. Noel-Baker was addressing a topic central to the then-current public discourse that was so much a part of everyday life during the Cold War era: the nuclear arms race. By the end of the evening, Lown was inspired; global nuclear war, he knew, would cause such environmental destruction that it would make the planet unlivable.

Lown and a few colleagues began holding biweekly meetings in his home to discuss what could be done and what they could offer as physicians. Finally, the doctors around Lown's table—pragmatists accustomed to the rigors of the scientific method, differential diagnosis, and peer-reviewed journals—decided to prepare a series of articles addressing the gruesome consequence to public health of a nuclear explosion. It was the dawn of a movement that would coalesce into

Physicians for Social Responsibility and would later expand across the world to meet new challenges in the 1980s as International Physicians for the Prevention of Nuclear War (IPPNW).

Their conclusions were published in a series of articles in the *New England Journal of Medicine*. Their conclusion, couched in data, was grim: Ultimately, Lown believed, modern medicine had nothing to offer victims of a nuclear war, "not even a token benefit."[4] The *New England Journal* articles—published as a symposium titled "The Medical Consequences of Thermonuclear War" on May 31, 1962—telegraphed the urgent message to physicians and researchers around the world.[5]

The articles drew the attention of the US military, Lown says, "and we thought the military would clobber us," saying, essentially, Who are you to speak with authority on a topic you know so little about? Instead, Lown says, the doctors received a request for reprints from the Pentagon. "The military sent an assistant secretary of defense to Boston to negotiate with us about our becoming expert consultants for the military. It proved essentially that doctors could make a substantial contribution to the nuclear debate."[6]

Doctors, Lown said, were well equipped by training and background to rise above dangerous stereotyping. They began to think of Russians as fellow human beings. "We made a break in the frozen thinking of how to diminish and start a journey backward in terms of nuclear weapons. We called it the medical prescription. Instead of negotiations among specialists in secret conclaves, which produced nothing except more weapons and more instability. . . . [W]e said, 'Let's begin with action.' This is medical common sense."[7] In 1979, after the accident at the Three Mile Island nuclear power plant in Pennsylvania, Lown wrote to a Russian acquaintance, Dr. Yevgeny Chazov, suggesting that Soviet and American doctors band together to oppose nuclear war. Lown and his colleagues got three hundred thousand children to write postcards to Ronald Reagan and Leonid Brezhnev, demanding the right to grow up and elicited one million petitions for disarmament and peace from other doctors.

By 1985, after numerous meetings, rallies, and colloquia, the two physicians—Lown of Boston and Chazov of Moscow—were awarded the Nobel Peace Prize.

Sometimes all it takes is one decision by one doctor to usher in a new era of research and innovation. If Alzheimer's seems like an opaque and impenetrable challenge with a potentially staggering caseload, perhaps some lessons can be drawn from the early days of the AIDS epidemic, more than a quarter-century ago. One young doctor, Anthony

Fauci, who was trained both in internal medicine and in immunology and infectious diseases, made a pioneering decision in the summer of 1981 that would turn his life around and engender a significant contribution to research on AIDS, which has become a global scourge. Looking back from the vantage point of the history of AIDS epidemiology over the past twenty-nine years, the impact Fauci made can be seen with more clarity. Now the director of the US National Institute of Allergy and Infectious Disease, he continues to work on the front lines of research into infectious diseases, and still focuses on AIDS.

In a telephone interview from his office, Fauci recalls the summer of 1981—June 5, to be exact—when he read about a small group of patients who had contracted an unusual strain of pneumonia. The report, in the *Morbidity and Mortality Weekly Report* (*MMWR*) of the national Centers for Disease Control, detailed the cases of five gay men in Los Angeles who developed Pneumocystis carinii pneumonia (PCP). "I was struck that pneumocystis pneumonia just doesn't occur in normal, healthy people. I said, wow, this is interesting, these young men must be immunosuppressed. But why the heck would they be immunosuppressed?"[8]

He put the *MMWR* aside and moved on to other matters. A month later, on July 4, he read another issue of the *MMWR* and found that there were twenty-six gay men from Los Angeles, San Francisco, and New York City who had PCP and a rare skin cancer called Kaposi's sarcoma. That report caught his attention: In fact, he says now, he has a vivid memory of sitting at his desk, saying, "Oh, my God," and getting goosebumps. "I've seen everything in medicine because even though I was quite young at the time, I had been very active in research in clinical medicine, and I had been seeing a lot of sick patients during the previous nine years. I knew that this was a new disease, that it had to be an infection, and that it had to be sexually transmitted. I couldn't figure out what it was. . . . Was it a mutation of cytomegalovirus? I just didn't know, nor did anybody else know."

Fauci had been intrigued his whole professional life by the human immune system. "Researchers for years had been working on mouse and guinea pig and rat and rabbit immunology," he says. "But we were just starting to make the transition into studying the human immune system. From the time I finished my fellowship and residency training in 1972, for about nine years, I was rather successful in building up a relatively prominent career for a young person at the time. So I was quite involved in what I was doing. As I tell people when I talk about what influences one's career: It is preparation and training and smarts, but it is also events beyond your control that shape what you do in life, not only professionally but probably personally and otherwise."

The patient Fauci was treating, thirty-six-year-old Ronald Resio of Alexandria, Virginia, succumbed to Pneumocystis carinii in August 1983, after undergoing bone marrow transplants and being treated with the experimental drug Interleukin-2. Fauci approached clinical puzzles with intellectual ferocity, weighing studies and clinical results, probing and questioning. Fauci's ultimate plan was to give patients several different treatments. Looking back, he recalls that his intuition told him the disease would not stay confined to the gay population. "I said to myself, you know, I've been trained as an infectious disease person, I've been trained as an immunologist, and my intuition tells me that this is going to be very much like hepatitis. It's blood-borne, it's sexually transmitted, and if it is sexually transmitted we are foolish to think that it's going to stay confined to the gay population. This is going to be a major pandemic." Six months later, researchers began to see the disease spread: the first cases of intravenous drug users suffering from a similar cluster of diseases began to be reported.

It was early fall of 1981 when Fauci made his decision: "I said, guess what, I'm going to change the direction of my research and I'm going to start bringing in these young men—and it was 99 percent gay men at the time—and study the abnormality of their immune system and try to figure out what it is that they have. Because I think this is going to explode, and I think this is not only potentially tragic but an exciting and an interesting field."

Fauci brought in two others to help with the clinical work; with that core of three people, the first HIV group at the National Institutes of Health was formed. His mentors and friends wondered exactly what he was doing, changing directions to study a bizarre disease that so far had been seen only in a handful of gay men. Fauci replied that even if the disease did afflict only gay men, it was still an important phenomenon deserving of study.

"And that's what I did," he says now. "From the end of the fall and the beginning of the winter of 1981–1982, I began admitting these patients, and the first several years were very bleak because all of our patients died. But we made some seminal observations in those early years about what the nature of the immune defect is. That really became very important in understanding the nature of the disease, [and was a factor] in the development of drugs and the development of vaccines."

As AIDS began to be seen in other continents, sickening heterosexual populations, particularly in Africa, the hunger for an accessible vaccine has deepened. In an article for *Nature* in May 2008, looking back at the twenty-five years since the human immunodeficiency virus was isolated in 1983, Fauci wrote that "much remains to be accomplished in the global fight against HIV." Cutting-edge drugs came into the market in the mid-1990s (protease inhibitors, which fight retroviruses like HIV, appeared in late 1995), and the AIDS death rate in the United States began to fall.

"The new therapies used in combination with older medicines rapidly improved the prognosis for vast numbers of HIV-infected patients," Fauci wrote. But, ever the analytical researcher, he added a caveat: "But HIV/AIDS is predominantly a disease of the developing world, where access to scientific advances and therapies is difficult."[9] Treatment alone is not a sufficient answer to a global pandemic. Programs that emphasize harm reduction and prevention—such as the distribution of condoms and clean needles—will be necessary, he says. And the major goal of research—a safe vaccine—is still elusive.

It is an incredible story in many ways, Fauci says. It is also the story of the impact one physician—who combined passion, intuition, and scientific rigor—made on one of the most significant emergent diseases in the twentieth century.

"It's not only the science, which was breathtaking in terms of the advances that we made. But also, the pharmaceutical companies were very motivated to make drugs, because they knew there would be millions and millions of people who would be taking a drug every day for the rest of their lives. At the end of the day, you need the pharmaceutical companies to be motivated to try and develop new drugs. It's no accident that we have more drugs for HIV than the sum total for all other drugs for all other viral diseases combined," he says. (Twenty-six individual drugs and four drug combinations had been approved by the FDA for HIV at the beginning of 2009.)

"I think I helped provide the momentum early on. In those early years, I did things that turned off a lot of people. And that doesn't mean other diseases are not equally as important, but I was able to say that this is something that is exploding in front of our eyes and we've got to do something about it. At the end of the day, I was right. It's all about getting up front, getting out there despite criticism and saying, 'Hey folks, this is going to be a major, global pandemic. We have got to address it.'"

New philosophical perspectives go from the hospice movement and the concept of palliative care to Physicians for Human Rights (PHR), which was a corecipient of the Nobel Peace Prize in 1997 for its work to ban landmines. We will likely soon see physician organizations devoted to environmental issues—if they do not exist already—because failure to heed the signs of climate change is a major threat to human health.

REAPPRAISING THE PROBLEM OF COGNITION IN ELDERS

Failure to attend to cognitive health and disregard for cognitive problems is a threat to human health. The underlying reasoning of organizations such as IPPNW, PHR, and others is that many social, political, and economic issues bear upon human health. The cognitive health of elders is a key component of global health concerns. Our societal attitude toward cognitive impairment is completely out of line with the system we have established to address the problem. Families are faced with fragmented services, disinterested doctors and hospitals, the ghettoizing of elders in nursing homes, inappropriate use of medications, inadequately trained physicians, and a payer system that rapidly impoverishes families.

The few solutions now on the table are Band-Aids that do not fundamentally change our thinking about caring for those with dementia and delaying its onset. The core rethinking for achieving lifelong cognitive health is directed toward lifestyle. Lifestyle adjustment is the only intervention we know about that can affect Alzheimer's disease. *There is no medication available now or expected to be available in the short-term future that can equal the effects of reducing lifestyle risk factors.* Every day we must make hundreds of decisions about our lifestyle—what to eat, whether to exercise, and so on—and all have medical consequences. But few doctors pay more than token lip service to the importance of these decisions. The medical model dictates that physicians ignore this area rather than create an arena in which the stakes are better understood.

On the one hand, the scale of these problems requires systemic restructuring as much as a shift in thinking. Proponents of radical change would like to see the existing system undergo controlled disassembly to create room for change. Although top-down social engineering is not an effective method for change, decisive action is needed for handling cognitive impairment in elders now and in the next decade as the ranks of the elderly swell. The system is stretched beyond capacity and is focused on inappropriate questions.

Medicine assumes the self-assured posture that all scientific knowledge is encompassed by the model. But scientific information is not uniform in its quality; what are considered "facts" rest upon vastly different levels of certainty. Here is how it works: Say you suspect drinking coffee protects you against Alzheimer's disease. So you set up a study and you find that those who drink coffee get Alzheimer's disease just as frequently as those who do not. This type of finding is called *absence of evidence*. So we discard the idea that coffee is either protective or harmful.

But wait a minute—not so fast. Suppose it turns out that those who drank more than two cups a day were protected or those who drank a special Colombian blend were protected or another, larger study came along that showed protection. One can name myriad additional factors that might suggest we hold the reins on any hasty conclusion. While absence of evidence is not evidence of absence, it can work the other way as well: coffee might seem protective for equally flimsy reasons.

Drawing conclusions about diet, as well as supplements and lifestyle, is extremely challenging. Likewise, drawing conclusions about pharmaceutical products with regard to their safety and efficacy carries staggering costs because achieving statistical significance requires large numbers of people who are stratified according to the numerous ways in which we differ from each other. Statistical significance alone is no guarantee that we are on the right track. In less politically correct times, statistics has been compared to clothing—it is what you *don't* see that is most interesting. One facet of the statistic we often do not see when a product is touted as beneficial is *how beneficial*. Suppose you don't like coffee or cannot afford the special recommended blend. Perhaps the benefit is so small that agonizing over a minuscule boost is not worth the effort.

As one looks deeper at a conclusion about health, the number of possible variables grows exponentially. How do other dietary factors or education or sleep patterns combine with coffee drinking to make an impact on Alzheimer's disease risk? How many years of coffee drinking are required to get effects—and starting at what age do you need to drink that coffee, and for how long? Does coffee prevent the disease or slow its progression? In general, investigators test one hypothesis at a time, and therefore cannot show how multiple factors work together in our complex lifestyles.

The frustration we feel about shifting views on dietary measures and disease risk is due to the impossibility of stratifying any study to capture the unique details of individual circumstances. Hypotheses are tested one at a time on imperfect sample populations and the results strung together with the assumption that if one treatment or risk factor is true, then two, three, or more treatments all together are also true. The scientific techniques used to test multiple interventions simultaneously require inconceivably large numbers of people to account for the huge number of variables in our lives. Ultimately we hit a conundrum because differences among broad-based population groups eventually reach the individual—each truly unique individual. And no study can generate statistical information with a sample size of one.

THE MEDICAL MODEL WILL NOT WORK IN THE COMING GENETIC REVOLUTION

The nascent field of personalized medicine attempts to reconcile the challenge of individual human differences with a statistical mean that blurs all differences into a single value. Personalized medicine improves upon decisions that have been based on a statistical mean by identifying the differences that predict one's individual risk for disease, and, in some cases, predict response to medications so that treatment can be tailored specifically for the individual.

One measure of human differences lies in snippets of DNA sequences that uniquely define an individual. No other person on the planet has exactly the same collection of small differences, or polymorphisms, as another, except in the case of identical twins. Each polymorphism is a place in the genome where the specific nucleotide—either an A, T, G, or C—can differ among individuals. If we numbered each of the three billion nucleotides—the A, T, G, Cs—of the human genome, giving each position in the genome a numeric value, we might find that a particular site tends to be an A, G, or C among various populations, but a T may have never been observed at that particular position. So if the polymorphic position we just described is usually an A, some people may have a G or a C in that same position.

For example, in scanning the long linear stretches of DNA, one might come across a place where most people have a T, but a small number of people from a certain geographic region or from a certain ethnic group tend to have a G. This polymorphism is a footprint of a historical event that occurred around the time when the geographic region first became populated or at the origin of a particular ethnic group. The descendants of the first person in whom the polymorphism occurred came to dominate the population numerically. Technically this phenomenon is called *fixation*, that is, the polymorphism became fixed in the population.

Millions of these ancient genetic events stud the genome, each carrying an untold story of mating and survival. Together, these polymorphisms are all that remain of the collection of stories that uniquely define an individual's past.

What makes polymorphisms of medical interest is that some of them increase the risk for disease. When a polymorphism results in a disease or increases the risk for a disease, we tilt toward using the term *mutation*, a word that carries the connotation that we know something about the consequences of the nucleotide change. So we might say a mutation is deleterious, beneficial, or even neutral if it has no consequences. Polymorphisms refer to the collection of all observed changes at a particular position in the genome, whether we know something about their consequences or not. And certainly we know nothing about the consequences of most of the millions of human polymorphisms. As we discussed in chapter 1 with regard to the presenilin gene, a small number of mutations are clearly deleterious. An even smaller number are clearly beneficial. And most changes in the DNA sequence from individual to individual have little or no consequence.

As we learn more about each polymorphism, some may predict a beneficial response to a medication, while others may predict side effects. Taking into account the functional consequences of the individual's gene mutations when prescribing a treatment program is a kind of personalized medicine, and it is clear that personalized medicine does not fit well with current practice. First, physician retraining will be necessary because most MDs lack knowledge of the genetics necessary for the interpretation of DNA tests. An even bigger obstacle is the one-size-fits-all philosophy of Big Pharma. Many companies prefer to develop drugs that will be useful to everyone and downplay individual differences. Personalized medicine offers an approach to tailor drugs for individuals with certain polymorphisms, and in so doing, to reduce side effects and increase efficacy. But the cost is losing those customers who do not have the indicated polymorphism. Big Pharma, logically, prefers to capture a larger customer base. The Vioxx debacle may have led some segments of Pharma to rethink the one-size-fits-all paradigm. This medication, manufactured by Merck, was prescribed to as many as 80 million people at one point, mainly for the treatment of arthritic pain, but was withdrawn from the market because a small number of patients had heart attacks associated with taking the drug. A more precise targeting of this drug to specific individuals might have safely salvaged a medication that was able to relieve pain in a large number of people.

The obstacles to meshing genetics with the medical model involve training doctors to be more knowledgeable about genetics; training a cadre of non-MDs who are comfortable talking about genetics with patients, families, and at-risk individuals; and creating viable economic structures for the implementation of personalized medicine without the stratospheric costs of the concierge doctor. Such doctors do not take insurance but instead charge patients a large, set fee per year in exchange for nearly unlimited attention. The concierge doctor may treat an elite, wealthy set of patients, but he or she usually does not know genetics either. The new personal genome companies are a response by the commercial sector to the abdication of genetics by the medical profession. The torpid nature of the medical profession, with its fear of technology (does your doctor communicate with you by e-mail?) has been caught unprepared by companies that offer online determination of your polymorphisms that put you at risk for many different diseases. All you do is send some spit in a special container to companies like 23andMe, or Navigenics; pay between a few hundred and a few thousand dollars (depending on the company and the services offered); and log into your personal genome site—and your computer screen becomes a genie that predicts your medical fate.

The *New England Journal of Medicine* as well as various medical associations have editorialized against direct-to-consumer genetic services. They point to the need for guidelines on the use of tests, standards for laboratory practice, accreditation of laboratories, ethical risks such as genetic discrimination, implications for family members, and privacy. The countervailing view is that individuals have the right to explore their own genome and should not be denied access, and [those who do restrict access are considered paternalistic. Lawmakers too have been caught in a quandary. In 2008, officials at the New York State Department of Health, in California, and in the Council of Europe attempted to legislate these companies by requiring a physician intermediary to deliver the genetic information to a client. Remember: genetic information is hot stuff with the potential to indicate erroneous conclusions and create enormous anxiety if you get bad news. And just about everybody has some bad news in their genes.

The results of genetic testing come as an alphabet soup of gene names attached to some risk for a disease, and the decision algorithm each company uses to assign a specific risk may be based on studies that vary widely in reproducibility. In other words, there is a reliability factor that is not revealed to the client. There's no getting around that— it's more a question of how much information you want and what level of information you need before you decide to take action. A 2008 editorial in *Nature Biotechnology* rather cynically summed up the regulatory argument as follows: "On balance, the argument goes, it is preferable for people to remain ignorant about their personal genome than to let the 'genome' out of the bottle."

This editorial goes on to say, "[T]he real concern is that many of the present objections overlook the vast scale of the challenge facing healthcare in the coming decades. It is virtually impossible to conceive of a sustainable form of healthcare that operates as the current systems in industrialized nations do. At present, healthcare is based on the late diagnosis of disease and the division of diseases into a few categories based on some overarching gross similarities. And it firmly places physicians as the central gatekeepers of information."[10]

This nugget of good sense captures the problem perfectly. Personalized medicine, based on individual rather than population data, with all its promise for improving efficacy of treatment and reducing side effects, will require that we intervene before the disease strikes. Our dependence on medical gatekeepers, whether they are physicians or genetic counselors, is misplaced and ultimately unaffordable. A genetic counselor at the personal genome company Navigenics told me that the most common action taken by the company's clients after receiving genomic data is to call their physician. If we are to spark a genetic revolution, we need greater access to credible and validated online data before we turn to the medical professional. The medical professional needs to be as comfortable with genetic data as he would be if he received a report from a highly specialized consultant. The physician then can help in the implementation of recommendations based on the genetic data—and hopefully prevent disease.

AT THE BOUNDARIES OF THE MEDICAL MODEL

Much of what we need to know about our health falls outside the medical model. The twin pillars of the profession are (on the medical side) drugs and (on the surgical side) the knife. When treatment involves neither drugs nor surgery, the problem falls outside the model. The typical nonmedical, nonsurgical treatments have been pushed to the fringes of healthcare. Herbal remedies, aromatherapy, yoga, reiki, holistic medicine, and just about any treatment not administered by a physician are sneered upon by the medical profession. The given reason for the disdain is lack of evidence of efficacy in double-blind crossover studies—essentially the standard for drug approval at the FDA. Ironically, this rigorous standard does not apply to new surgical procedures. Surgeons can do pretty much what they please in the operating room. Folk medicine and alternative medicine have some credibility based on their long use in certain cultures, but they lack scientific validation, so pinning one's hopes for a cure on alternative medicine represents an unknown risk. Without a billion-dollar pharmaceutical pot of cash behind them, nonpharmacological treatments such as massage, exercise, meditation, and many others can never reach the same standard of scientific rigor. And if these approaches did reach the same standard, they are not protected by a patent and therefore hold no attraction to the industry.

Pinning one's hopes for a cure on an approved pharmaceutical solution is also a percentage game. However, compared to folk remedies and alternative medicine, there is more formal knowledge about what the percentages are for the success of medications. Few, if any, drugs are 100 percent effective; most fall far below that mark. The likelihood of developing side effects is also a percentage game. An effective medical encounter requires some understanding of probability and how to weight probabilities. Treatments backed by data must be weighed against treatments backed only by anecdotal information or informal information because there has been no clinical trial. Few doctors present the nuances of the entire picture weighed against the individual needs of the patient in front of them.

So what do you want from your doctor? You'd like to know the effectiveness and risk of FDA-approved drugs for your condition. You'd like to know what other options are out there, especially if the approved drugs are not working or if the side effects are intolerable. You'd like to know how nonpharmacologic measures might help your condition, perhaps in conjunction with pharmaceutical approaches. Most of this information you will not get from your doctor—and in fact, you will often not get from any reliable source. Instead, you will be forced to guess what facets of your condition or what treatments fall within the interests of the doctor, seeking answers and help elsewhere for whatever lies outside the medical model. You must tread gingerly over queries about nonmedical approaches because the physician might cursorily dismiss the question entirely or launch into some tangential response that consumes precious minutes of contact time. In the absence of good information sources, you might turn to a vendor behind the counter at the local health food store whose credentials are unknown, someone motivated only by selling his products. Many health food stores have recognized this knowledge gap, and some of their employees are highly articulate about supplements and nutriceuticals. However, when pushed a bit for supporting data about the claims he is making, he usually comes up empty—and the charming vendor might become less than cordial.

APPLICATION OF THE MEDICAL MODEL
TO CONDITIONS THAT AFFECT THE MIND

Alzheimer's disease straddles the line between mental and physical illness. While the clinical symptoms of Alzheimer's disease fall well within the realm of conditions described in psychiatry manuals—such as paranoia, impulsivity, depression, and hallucinations, among others—the disease has a strong physical basis in the brain. The senile plaques and neurofibrillary tangles are easily visible diagnostic hallmarks. Patient advocates hold onto those physical traces like a life raft, because without them, patients would be cast adrift in a murky sea of highly stigmatized mental diseases. Even family members of the mentally ill can be stigmatized, being blamed for causing the illness. Caregivers and family members may have their own mental health status questioned, or be rejected by relatives and friends. It seems like a trick we play on our minds to feel greater empathy for a suffering individual who has a microscopically visible structure in her brain than we do for someone who is suffering equally but is lacking a physical marker.

Alzheimer's disease is a condition in which the damage to the brain—the plaques and tangles—concomitantly destroys the mind. As it is a disease with mostly psychiatric symptoms but that also has physical underpinnings, application of the medical model faces a duality. Among the vocal critics of applying the medical model to conditions that affect the mind are rebels, skeptics, and freethinkers who have all played upon the uncertainties and intangibles we call the mind, questioning the validity of extending our approaches from diseases of the body to diseases of the mind. For example, Thomas Szasz claimed in his libertarian treatises that mental illness was just a metaphor used by those who want to oppress others, and R. D. Laing saw some mental conditions as a preferred perspective on reality. But as the brain fills up with plaques and tangles that squeeze out the complex brain circuitry of the individual's mental life, there is not even the remotest possibility that the Alzheimer's patient suffers from a metaphor conjured up by oppressors or from a preferred perspective on reality.

But not all criticism of the medical model has been misguided. A more sociologically based critique of the medical model came from Ivan Illich, who wrote in his 1975 book *Medical Nemesis* about the overmedicalization of health issues.[11] Illich wanted to aim the focus of medicine toward disease prevention and elimination rather than placing people into life-long roles as patients. As a patient, according to Illich, one is subject to a further decline in health because the patient role calls for the patient to be sick. Although people are generally not consciously inclined to prolong their role as a patient, the pathway out of the grasp of the medical profession is beset with traps. Nosocomial infections acquired in hospitals, iatrogenic diseases caused by the treatment itself, medical errors, and drug side effects are all dangers that conspire to prolong our role as patient and make us wary of the medical system. Similarly, the preferred treatment option among pharmaceutical companies is a pill a day for the rest of one's life. Eradication of a disease does not make for the best business model. Most people simply accept that a chronic disease like Alzheimer's will require daily treatment. Unfortunately, the research enterprise does not yet know how to slow the course of Alzheimer's with chronic drug administration, or how to eradicate the disease.

In 1961, more than a decade before *Medical Nemesis*, Erving Goffman in *Asylum* described the acculturation of inmates and keepers to a set of rules that socialized them to their roles. Ken Kesey fictionalized Goffman's sociological studies in his novel *One Flew over the Cuckoo's Nest* in 1975. An acculturation process also occurs with Alzheimer patients. The process is first an adaptation to the medical model that addresses relatively few aspects of the complexities of the disease and later involves acculturation within a facility that in some cases does not seem to have advanced very far beyond the asylums described by Goffman and Kesey. Nursing homes thus join asylums, monasteries, prisons, the army, and orphanages as "total institutions," closed off from the world with every aspect of daily life controlled.

APPLICATION OF THE MEDICAL MODEL TO CONDITIONS THAT AFFECT THE BRAIN

The modern tertiary-care hospital, often called a "medical center" in recognition of its growing territorial claims, stands like a temple in which the rules of the medical model are most strictly practiced. The entry criteria to the medical sanctum is to pull out all stops and attempt to cure whatever ails a patient—no matter how unrealistic, no matter how costly, and no matter how invasive. Once a condition is recognized as incurable or no longer amenable to medical intervention, or if the patient loses interest in what is offered, the hospital enterprise backs away and seeks to discharge the person to a vast, unruly morass of institutions and facilities designed to accept those with medical conditions that persist outside the temple. Such individuals must travel an uncharted route often far outside the mainstream.

With the medical model comes a certain degree of bravado. Deciding that a frail gentleman in his eighties needs an operation—with all the attendant risks of surgery and no certainty of benefit—requires the kind of confidence for which surgeons are well known. No one is there to weigh the obvious conflict of interest: surgery, whether beneficial or not, enriches the coffers of both surgeon and hospital. Not surprisingly, the surgeons, whose very job description requires a rosy outlook for all comers, sit atop the income ladder in hospitals. Next on the ladder are those physicians who directly support the surgeons: the radiologists and the anesthesiologists. Physicians who simply talk to patients without doing any procedures—the psychiatrists—sit at the bottom of the income ladder. Because patients turn to physicians who claim their interventions will work—why do otherwise?—physicians have a great incentive to spin the patient's condition overoptimistically. Few people want to go to a doctor who says, "I'm sorry, the chances of my treatment working are negligible." And patients rail against doctors who tell them their condition is terminal. That is not to say that patients want their doctor to deceive them, but at some level people do prefer a pleasant deception to a grim truth.

Nevertheless, at some point the medical options run out, and regardless of the doctor's compassion, the medical enterprise loses interest. The medical model is not geared toward all people with illnesses—it is geared only toward those people with illnesses that can be treated within the medical system. Furthermore, it is geared only toward those people who can be treated within the medical system in a cost-effective manner—meaning that the patient can afford the treatment and the hospital can afford to provide the treatment. Everyone is aware of the large percentage of the US population who cannot afford medical services. But less recognized is the large percentage of the population that is not adequately treated *regardless of their financial situation* because the multibillion-dollar medical system has abandoned them. Filling the gap, in their modern stripes, continue to be mystics, witches, *curanderos*, and spiritualists to satisfy the desperate longing for a cure. When disease strikes, our vulnerability goes far beyond the infectious agent, the tumor cells, the clogged arteries, or any other pathology—our vulnerability leads us to suspend judgment and latch onto any thread of hope, no matter how futile.

Perhaps the largest population abandoned by the medical system is people with Alzheimer's disease. Just as in our communities, the best hospital real estate goes to the wealthy—the surgeons. Unlike cancer and heart disease, Alzheimer's disease never involves surgery, so patients with the disease are often relegated to the least desirable and most obscure space. Ironically, finding the location of the physicians who deal with Alzheimer's disease within a large medical center is challenging even for those whose minds are completely intact. Once the neurologist has completed her evaluation, other services are fragmented into care silos that are equally difficult to find, require long wait intervals between appointments, and have minimal communication among them. Rarely does anyone take a comprehensive view of the problems and make each visit efficient by having on hand all the necessary expertise in one place.

Once the diagnosis of Alzheimer's disease is made, most physicians—even neurologists—lose interest, mainly because they have little to offer. Certainly no procedures, which are the lucrative side of medicine, are indicated. But the needs and questions of the patient and family mount. Their concerns increasingly deviate from what falls within the medical model. The discussions become time consuming; the areas of concern move toward social, economic, and legal questions, areas in which physicians are not trained, not compensated, and not particularly interested. Yet often families continue to return to the doctor, adding to the frustration on both sides. The doctor has a cure mentality, which is much appreciated for a curable disease, of course. But there is a direct corollary here: medical practices that are focused on cure are not concerned with chronic, incurable diseases. The patient wants some attention to practical measures or information about research, neither of which can be provided by most physicians. To make matters worse, the considerable time required by dementia patients backs up the clinic, and soon the waiting room fills with disgruntled patients faced with long waits for their own appointments.

Since her mother was diagnosed with dementia of the Alzheimer's type in 2003, Dierdre Scanlan has somehow managed to maintain her footing.[12] By any account, it cannot be easy to weather the death of her father and the loss of a sibling, keep two children on track in school, and work full-time. But she draws on her own deep wellspring of humor and compassion, and occasionally invokes the spirit and never-surrender streak of her Irish forebears.

Dierdre's father was the planner in the family, the one who took care of the bills and organized vacations. So her mother, more passive by nature, was somewhat hard to diagnose. The family noticed that Barbara Scanlan had become more withdrawn, and she herself alluded to a feeling of something being wrong.

"So we went and talked to a neurologist for the first time, and they did a CT scan, an MRI. . . . [T]hey were looking to see if there had been some kind of brain damage or if there was pressure on the brain," she says. "All of those tests showed that she hadn't suffered head trauma and hadn't had a series of strokes. So they placed her on the [Alzheimer's] spectrum and started her on different medications."

Her mother started out on Aricept, which made her sick to her stomach, so she was switched to Namenda. "That did not seem to be helping, but it didn't seem to be hurting, either, so she stayed on that a good while," Dierdre says in an interview at an Irish pub in the greater Boston area. The most improvement seems to have come from Exelon, a cholinesterase inhibitor delivered in a twenty-four-hour patch. "It's not that Exelon has improved her memory, but she does not seem to be on such a roller coaster emotionally and she is not as anxious. She is just a little bit more even. I think it is probably from getting an even dose every twenty-four hours. But there has been a lot of flailing around and an enormous number of visits to doctors who are not neurologists, who said, 'Maybe it's not dementia, maybe there's something else going on.' There has been a lot of wasted time."

Dierdre's father, Jacob, who was in his eighties when he died, was able to take his wife to doctor's appointments until he himself became ill in the fall of 2008. But Dierdre, who works for a New York–based firm, still took the lead on researching tests and drugs and keeping current on recommended doctors; that work proved to be a part-time job in itself, so she reduced the hours she worked at her paying job. "My father was a very smart guy, and if I took the lead in saying, 'We need to get such-and-such a test,' he could bring her."

With two elderly parents and two children in school, Dierdre's weeks were a juggling act that required split-second timing. There was little time for her own medical appointments or tending to other personal business. She visited her parents, then still living in a house in a small town in Massachusetts, every Friday while her children were in school. Visits did not necessarily involve extensive conversations, either. On many days, it was enough to be present. Other times, she would bring books and articles about Alzheimer's for her parents, since they did not have a computer or Internet connection. She also took her parents to presentations on Alzheimer's at community hospitals in the area. "I'm not sure how much of it she was really taking in. It was more for my father than for her. Finally, Jacob joined an Alzheimer's support group at the senior center in the town where they lived. But I could see it was costing him more and more time, and that it was more and more difficult for him to do everything."

Jacob was happy to have his wife still living in the home they had built together, even though Barbara was not capable of performing the simplest domestic chores. She could no longer cook and could do very little cleaning. She still recognized her husband, daughters, grand-children, and sons-in-law, which her family found comforting. But when her husband died, she was confused: Where did he go? Did he really die? Did he not die, but leave in some other way? The death of her husband and her own increasing frailty meant Barbara had to be moved into assisted living. The four-bedroom family house, where the couple lived for fifty years and raised three children, is being sold. "She still is at the stage of learning things. You have to repeat things over and over, you have to reteach her things for a long time, but then she gets it. Now she knows that she is not living in her house, that we have moved her into assisted living. And she knows she has Alzheimer's. But she is utterly confused about lots of things."

Because the assisted living facility is only fifteen minutes away from her home, Dierdre checks in with her mother often and helps her shower. "I find myself half living over there. The staff members are very nice; they take her down for three meals a day. It's large, so we have someone who brings her down to the dining room and back because she is afraid of getting lost." But balancing her role as daughter, wife, and mother while doing research on the disease, keeping up with her mother's doctor's appointments, and visiting the assisted living facility can be wearing. "You feel a lot of guilt. This year it seems to be better than it has been before, because my kids [who are in high school] don't seem as needy." Dierdre reflects on her changed role in the family. "I'm the parent of the mother, and my husband is the parent of the kids. And you know, we all hit this stage. We're all having kids later, and our parents are old, they're in their eighties. Something is bound to happen."

Dierdre believes her mother's encroaching dementia went undiag-nosed for some time because Barbara always seemed to cope with a low level of depression. Barbara sees a neurologist for follow-ups and for medication, but, as Dierdre notes, there is not a lot that can be done to "stem the tide. You're basically going to them for maintenance." There is no timeline and no prognosis. "You tend to be trying to figure out your next move and all the while you're wondering, 'Is it really Alzheimer's or is it something else?' And unless my mother has one of those long-range cases of Alzheimer's that could take twenty years, you never know exactly where you are."

> There's that gap between a guy who is completely self-sufficient and the nursing home guy who was in bed 90 percent of the time staring at a fuzzy TV screen. In that gap, in the space between the two points, there's a need for some help. It would have been nice to be able to keep him at home. Nowadays families are all over the place now, not like fifty or sixty years ago where everybody is living in the same house. Everybody has their own lives, so the care really falls on the spouse, who often has their own problems. You need help.
>
> —BENNO FALCONE

Gennaro Falcone's symptoms were subtle at first. A self-made businessman in a tight-knit Italian neighborhood in a city on the East Coast, he shouldered his way to prosperity. His son Benno acquired the Ivy League polish his father dreamed of, along with a law degree. When the old man retired, however, Benno saw changes. "He had retired in his early seventies, and he was long retired before we noticed the symptoms and changes," Benno says. "He wasn't able to do the tasks he was able to do easily in the past. He'd make a point of coming over and helping me—plumbing, electrical projects. He was an all-around capable guy, and we noticed he was losing those capabilities. It would frustrate him greatly."[13]

Although a brother lived next door, the family worried that the arguments between their parents were growing more heated. Gennaro would lash out verbally. Benno's mother, Julia, although increasingly frail, would respond in kind. "Up until the last year or so, she was able to handle him, to deal with him. Of course, personality-wise, they would clash. She's ninety now, but they're old-timers. My mother is rough around the edges. She knew what was happening and nonetheless it had an impact on her; she had difficulty adjusting. They would clash and argue. She's not the kind of person that would—well, what's on her mind is on her lips." Every now and again, Benno says, he and his brothers would pay a visit and referee the battle.

A sister, Stacia, moved in to take care of both parents. But Gennaro's physical deterioration accelerated. Once robust, he became unsteady on his feet. He couldn't plan his day. He went to the bathroom whenever he wanted to, regardless of the setting. Although the family kept him close and included him in every aspect of their lives, outings were embarrassing. "One time, I took him down to the boat, we were walking down the dock and I gave him a small task to keep him busy," Benno says. "He was helping me wrap up a hose or something like that, and he had difficulty with it. Then he disappeared. He went to the end of the dock because he had to go to the bathroom. He really started to lose his inhibitions and judgment in the last year."

Gennaro knew at some level that a void was approaching. He had difficulty driving, missing turns and forgetting how to get home. He stopped socializing with friends, which isolated his wife and sparked more arguments. "When you did go out," Benno says, "it just wasn't worth it. The last several years, it was like taking a toddler with you, making sure he went to the bathroom and did not get into trouble."

When Gennaro became too hot to handle at home, the family enrolled him at a day program affiliated with a local senior center. But most of the patients were sedentary and infirm, either mentally or physically. "My father was not sedentary," Benno says. "He'd want to get up and do things and go places, so he didn't mix well with their routine. He'd leave [the day program] and they'd call the police and the police would come take my father back. My father would say, 'What are you doing? What am I doing here with these people? I have things to do at home in the yard.'"

Things got better when the family enrolled Gennaro in a specialized day program in a light-filled home that kept patients active with daily walks, music and art therapy, and the opportunity to interact with staff and with other patients. It wasn't perfect, but it seemed to fill Gennaro with purpose. "In terms of dealing with people with this disease, it's an area that's lacking," Benno says. "Whether it be daycare or nursing homes, [good ones] are few and far between. We have to recognize that society is not in the position to afford it all, but I've found in the last couple of months that most of these nursing homes are trained to deal with people in a semivegetative state. They are ill, but peaceful."

Toward the end, as his father slid toward death, Benno found a full-time nursing home. And although he understood the need for heavy sedation because his father was so agitated, he was tormented. "Sometimes I went to the nursing home to visit him near the end and they had him medicated so much he was barely conscious. It got to a point where in the last several months you began to think that the end would be a blessing for him."

What would he change, if he could? "For the average person—and I think we are average people—getting enough help to be able to get the assistance necessary to keep him at home. I guess if you're a millionaire and money is no object, [you] can hire a full-time nurse with specialized training to stay around the clock. But near the end, his needs changed." That, Benno says, is the precise location of the care gap: between part-time home health aides and day programs, and full-time nursing home care. "There didn't seem to be a lot of options available for assistance in that period of time. That is the biggest frustration, I think, beyond the frustrations of dealing with it emotionally. It's different from most diseases, where you lose somebody and there is a grieving period. With [Alzheimer's], there is a gradual loss, you are losing a person, and then you still have the grieving period when you lose him completely."

The problem of Alzheimer's disease is actually abandoned by the medical profession long before people even get the disease. Effective measures to delay the onset of Alzheimer's are known, and yet the medical profession has no comprehensive Alzheimer's prevention program. The reason? Prevention falls outside the medical model and is therefore not reimbursable. As the conversation with your doctor turns from prescription drugs to supplements, diet, exercise, or cognitive remediation, just watch his expression grow impatient. It will become rapidly apparent that his interest level is plummeting. The medical model draws a sharp line with regard to what lies in its armamentarium and what does not. But the line that divides what helps people and what does not is much less sharp. In a moment, one can slip away from the legitimate world of medicine and fall into what medicine views as the kooky fringe of herbal compounds, acupuncture, and meditation; and once on this slippery slope it's only another small step to shamans and sorcerers. But medicine's disdain for measures that are neither drugs nor surgery occludes a wide terrain of really helpful interventions that get tossed out with the shamans and sorcerers. So-called alternative medicine remedies are of interest to vast numbers of people. Such remedies are of particular interest to people with an incurable disease as are equally unknown remedies that are tested in clinical trials. For therapies that fall outside the medical model advice, even advice about their safety, the doctor is mum, and for research therapies the doctor is usually ignorant. There is no easy way to guide patients on what research studies are available, what research is suited for them, and what unresearched approaches might offer some salve for the unbearable burden of watching one's own identity vanish.

As we proceed in our thinking about these issues and possible solutions, I hope it will become apparent that we can do a lot better. We can deliver care more effectively, we can better inform patients and families, we can implement programs that will reduce the numbers of Alzheimer patients—and we can do all of this in a cost-effective manner. Most

5

THE ALZHEIMER BURDEN
AND THE COMING EPIDEMIC

The old doctor felt my pulse, evidently thinking of something else
the while. "Good, good for there," he mumbled, and then with a
certain eagerness asked me whether I would let him measure my
head. Rather surprised, I said Yes, when he produced a thing like
calipers and got the dimensions back and front and every way,
taking notes carefully. He was an unshaven little man in a thread-
bare coat like a gaberdine, with his feet in slippers, and I thought
him a harmless fool. "I always ask leave, in the interests of science, to measure the crania of those going out there," he said.
"And when they come back, too?" I asked. "Oh, I never see
them," he remarked; "and, moreover, the changes take place
inside, you know."

—THE PROJECT GUTENBERG
HEART OF DARKNESS, BY JOSEPH CONRAD

The idea of living on our retirement income, a gauzy dream perpet-
uated by financial institutions, may always have rested someplace
between myth and reality. Now, with grim economic news swirling
nationwide, it has vanished for many. The simple formula offered by
financial advisers—plug your financial data into a program, enter the
amount of money you want during your retirement, and then cash the
check—was never all that simple, and never guaranteed. Baby boomers
have received an economic wake-up call: if they retire at all, it will be
when they are well into their sixties or even their seventies. And they

will still be working at an age when Alzheimer's disease strikes at ever-increasing rates. Taken together, this creates a demographic time bomb.

ALZHEIMER DISEASE BY THE NUMBERS

One might think about the coming epidemic of Alzheimer's disease like a resident of New Orleans might listen to a weather advisory about the threat of a hurricane in the Gulf aimed directly at the city. Unlike a hurricane, however, the chances of the Alzheimer epidemic veering off course are slim to none, enabling us to see the leading edge of the epidemic. Broadly mobilizing concern for the problem of Alzheimer's disease requires an accurate set of numbers that can reveal the magnitude of the problem. As of March 2007, more than five million people in the United States, or about 1.6 percent of the population, are living with Alzheimer's disease. This number represents a 10 percent increase over the estimate from the Alzheimer's Association five years earlier. We are seeing the leading edge of the epidemic.[1] Every seventy-two seconds, someone develops the disease. And the news gets worse: The number of Americans with Alzheimer's disease is expected to double over the next thirty years.

According to the US Census Bureau, there were an estimated 78.2 million American baby boomers (those born between 1946 and 1964) as of July 1, 2005.[2] Baby boomers began turning sixty at a rate of about 330 every hour in 2006, and by 2011, baby boomers will begin turning sixty-five, reaching the age of significant risk for Alzheimer's disease. Because the plaques and tangles begin a decade or two before symptoms, some people now in their forties are depositing in their brains the earliest of stigmata of Alzheimer's disease.

Of those reaching the traditional retirement age of sixty-five, 13 percent, or one in eight, have Alzheimer's disease, according to statistics compiled by the Alzheimer's Association. We are on track for an explosion of Alzheimer's disease as the baby boomers start turning sixty-five. Rates soar for those over eight-five, and Alzheimer's disease rises to the frighteningly large percentage of nearly half the population in this age bracket. According to the current trajectory, 7.7 million people will have the disease by 2030 and as many as sixteen million could be affected by 2050.[3]

While the at-risk pool for Alzheimer's disease are the aged, when aging is combined with some of the most common chronic diseases, such as cardiovascular disease or diabetes, the risk goes even higher. In

2000, the number of people with at least one chronic disease reached 125 million, at a cost of $510 billion, and these numbers will continue to grow to 160 million by 2020 at cost of $1 trillion. These combined conditions (approximately 2.4 chronic conditions) put older persons at risk for problems arising from taking many medications simultaneously, since each patient receives on average 5.1 prescriptions.

Collectively, the direct and indirect costs of Alzheimer's and other dementias amount to more than $148 billion annually. Medicare costs in 2005 were $91 billion, and in 2010 these costs will be $160 billion, or more than $530 per person. So a family of four is shouldering $2,120 yearly toward Medicare if the costs were distributed equally.[4]

Sadly, Alzheimer's disease strikes at a time when people may be looking forward to their retirement and a chance to do things they have postponed for decades. They may want to travel or spend more time with family or sort out a lifetime of remembrances boxed away in the basement or the attic. Often couples have worked hard to put aside savings for this time in their lives, but all those plans come skidding to a halt as a spouse's personality deteriorates. The plans are no longer feasible, the saved money needs to go for long-term care, and, for couples, their very relationship itself needs to be redefined.

Alzheimer's disease is an "equal opportunity disease" in the sense that with relatively minor variation the likelihood of getting the disease is similar in all cultures, all geographic locations, all ethnicities, and all socioeconomic groups. In the rare places where the prevalence of the disease is significantly higher, the cause is almost certainly due to a local clustering of risk factors. Conversely, if death at a young age is high in a given country, people there do not reach the point where they are at risk for dementia. Elsewhere, a condition such as very high blood pressure may be common, and the incidence of strokes with the associated cognitive decline may outpace Alzheimer's disease. Forty-three million adults have hypertension in the United States—including two-thirds of people over the age of sixty—and it is likely that all are at risk for Alzheimer's disease.

One exception to the "equal opportunity" rule is the disproportionate number of women affected by the disease: the incidence is greater, even when statisticians take into account the fact that women live longer than men. According to data from the venerable Framingham Heart Study, women have a one-in-six chance of developing Alzheimer's disease in their lifetime, while the risk for men is one in ten. (Begun in 1948, the Framingham Heart Study collected blood samples from two-thirds of the adult population of Framingham, Massachusetts. Follow-up exams, by Boston

University and the National Heart, Lung, and Blood Institute, have assessed the health of subsequent generations—and participants have been followed for a number of diseases, not just heart ailments.)[5] The lifetime risk of developing any dementia was more than one in five for women, and one in seven for men. To gather these statistics the researchers followed 2,794 dementia-free participants of the Framingham Heart Study for twenty-nine years. They found 400 cases of dementia of all types and 292 cases of Alzheimer's disease.

The basis for this difference is unknown. Given the same number of neurofibrillary tangles in a man or a woman, the woman tends to be more clinically impaired. This finding has led to the conclusion that women are more affected by the disease process, but again the physiological basis for this observation is unknown. The disease may also affect women differently than men. Women tend to have greater language deficits, are more reclusive and emotionally labile, often hoarded, refused help, and had inappropriate laughter or crying. Male patients exhibit greater abusiveness, aggression, social impropriety, and wandering, particularly in the more advanced stages of the disorder. Given these behavioral discrepancies, it is not surprising that major tranquilizers and behavior management programs are used more frequently on male patients.

INSTITUTIONALIZATION

Alzheimer's disease is the most frequent cause of institutionalization for long-term care.[6] Among the leading reasons why people put their loved ones into institutions is because the affected individual is unable to care for himself and the family cannot care for him. Families often use these terms to describe their decision: "I couldn't forgive myself if something happened," "It was ruining my life," and "I had no choice." Failure to attend to personal hygiene and personality disorders, even violence, are often the immediate proximate causes for "placement." Placement is one of those detached abstract terms used by the healthcare industry both to dehumanize and to neutralize the transition from one's home to a long-term care facility. It is hard to imagine a more painful life milestone. Sometimes it takes a film, or a novel, to convey the wrenching emotions elicited. *Away from Her*, directed by Sarah Polley with Gordon Pinsent, Stacey LaBerge, and Julie Christie, provides a close-up. (For those who wish to explore further, the film is based on a book by Alice Munro called *The Bear Came over the Mountain*.)[7]

One woman in the greater Boston area, whom we'll call Renée, struggled with the decision to put her father in a nursing home near her. As is true for many, the decisive moment came when her father began wandering around the neighborhood and could no longer keep up with his own personal hygiene. The family tried moving him in with one of his daughters, but the burden of finding homecare aides, while running a household with children, became overwhelming. Placing him was harder than she expected. "One nursing home we looked at actually wouldn't accept him because they said his dementia was not severe enough," says Renée. "There wasn't a floor [in the nursing home devoted to memory care] for him. He was not able to live alone and care for himself, but his dementia was not so severe, either."

While Renée has been happy with the level of care her father receives in the nursing home, gaps have inevitably appeared. "I wish they'd take better care of his things. His clothes and shoes get lost, his money gets lost. He's a man who likes to carry money, so now we give him Ones [dollar bills] to hold. It would be nice to make a request one time, and not to have to follow up on it. This must sound awful, but he refuses help from any person who is not Caucasian and who is female. He gets very embarrassed," Renée says. She adds that social factors can sometimes influence how a patient is treated. "I think if the patient has a lot of visitors, if the facility knows the family is involved, the staff will stay on their toes," she says. "I've called the Department of Public Health—and maybe someone might think this is trivial—because a dentist went in and pulled one of my father's teeth, the wrong tooth—without our permission. So there have been rocky times there, and pleasant times, too. You get to know the people you feel you can trust."

The emotional cost of "placement" has been high. "Well, they're housing them. They'll say, 'He's fine,' but nursing homes are not the nicest places to visit someone you adore. It's hard to see everyone else, sitting and waiting [to die]. I think emotionally when you put a parent into a nursing home, a corner of your heart breaks off."

The campus of Bright Ridge spills out along the highway in a former cornfield, surrounded by the big-box stores and chain restaurants that mark most American exurbs. It is the kind of elder complex that awaits most baby boomers—if they are lucky. Smartly decorated and well staffed, it offers apartments for those who are still independent enough to cook and get around by themselves; an assisted living wing for those who need some help; and a memory care unit for those who have dementia. Inside, Bright Ridge has re-created a small-town atmosphere that must be of some comfort to the residents, many of whom grew up on farms or in hamlets in rural regions of the Upper Midwest. Near the door, a flat-screen television scrolls through a list of activities for the day. There is a bank, a hair salon, and a small store with sundry items for sale. Residents traverse the corridors on foot, using canes and walkers, or perched on smart-looking electric scooters. A few visit with relatives, smiling at the antics of grandchildren. Others stare vacantly.

Jan Thorgaard ended up here unexpectedly. Jan was able to keep her husband, Harold, at home for a year after his diagnosis in 2000. They retired from their jobs and took a much-anticipated vacation together. But their time at home was not to last. Increasingly, Harold had difficulty managing the simple tasks of daily life, and it took all of Jan's energy to monitor him.

"It's such a lonely walk," she says. "You're tied to home, because you get to the point where you can't go out without them, but you can't go out with them. At the beginning, friends and family are supportive. But then, as time goes on, they don't know what to do or how to do it, or what to say."[8]

She discovered Bright Ridge, took a tour, and moved both of them into an apartment in the independent living wing of the complex. Harold continued to be seen from time to time by his primary-care physician, who could offer little beyond Aricept to delay the slide into dementia. As Harold's Alzheimer's progressed, Jan had to strategize constantly to stay one step ahead. Like many patients, Harold began to wander at night. After he walked outside the Bright Ridge building and got locked out, Jan installed a motion detector near the door to their apartment. She laughs, somewhat ruefully, as she recalls her husband's attempts to outwit the system. "He got to the point that he knew if he stood perfectly still, it wouldn't ring. He would walk into it and stand there for a while, and it would shut off. Then he would take a couple more steps, and he would stand there. If I didn't respond right away, he could get out the door. He got really tickled because I walked into it one morning when I got up. He thought that was very funny. You have to find humor in this, or else you couldn't make it."

Harold also retained some of his skills as a mechanic, and put them to use by taking the toilet apart during the night. "I got to the point where I duct-taped the top onto the toilet so he couldn't get in there," Jan says. "I could hear him get up at night, and I could hear that tape coming loose. I would get up and bring him back to bed. He did that when he went into memory care, too. Every room had its own bathroom. They would wander in and out of each other's rooms. . . . The staff would find him taking somebody's toilet apart. One of the gals finally cured it. She went

in there when she found him one day and she asked Harold if he had a license to be doing plumbing work. He said, no, he didn't have a license. She suggested he had better stop, and he never went back. He remembered that he had to have a license to do his air-conditioning and heating repair. They were quite good at treating him with respect, at meeting him where he was as the Alzheimer's progressed."

There came a point, Jan says, when she could no longer cope. She considered hiring an aide to come in, but ultimately decided that their apartment at Bright Ridge was too confining. So Jan Thorgaard made the hard decision to commit her husband to the memory care unit. "Believe me, that is the hardest decision anybody will ever make," she says. Although the unit was a few steps away from her apartment, although she visited every day, she could not help but mourn for their old life together. Harold died fifteen months later.

On another floor at Bright Ridge, Annette Edmonds recalls the whirlwind courtship that led to her second marriage—and the way that Alzheimer's disease brought an abrupt end to things.[9] In her eighties, she had been widowed long ago and had grown used to the single life. In fact, she relished it. She could still travel, and she was surrounded by scores of good friends. Then she got a phone call from Bill, an old friend from her married days. She hadn't kept up with him, but he quickly filled her in on the milestones in his life. He was a widower, and he wanted to move away from the East Coast and resettle. A westerner at heart, he had never been comfortable with the pace of life around the Beltway, near Washington, DC. In fact, he was thinking of moving nearby. Annette was surprised, but found herself talking to Bill by phone once or twice every day. He flew out for a visit, and both realized that their chemistry was genuine. They set a date to be married.

"He went back home to clean out his house, and we resumed talking every day by long distance. I thought he sounded very tired and a little confused, but I knew he had been working hard," Annette says. The next few months were busy. They wrote their vows and planned a marriage ceremony to be held in a small church. Annette picked out a dress and sent out invitations, and Bill moved into her apartment. The wedding was a touching blend of new possibility and nostalgia. Bill and Annette both have children, adults now, who walked them down the aisle. They were so exhausted from the wedding, however, that they delayed a honeymoon trip out west. Unfortunately, Bill never seemed to regain his old energy.

"The first thing I ever noticed was when we decided to move from our condo out to Bright Ridge. He was driving and he turned onto a

four-lane highway on the wrong side. I screamed and he pulled over."
Annette asked him to stop driving, but he demurred. Annette attributed
the wrong turn to exhaustion.

"One day he was doing his own income tax and I could see that he
was a little bit confused about it. He came to me one day with the
income tax report and said, 'Could you arrange these pages for me? I
can't seem to get them arranged.' They were all mixed up. They were
numbered, but he couldn't seem to put them in order." It was a troubling sign, she thought, for a man with a distinguished academic career
and a knack for numbers.

Then, anxiety and paranoia began to darken Bill's mood. He jeal-
ously guarded the contents of his desk and refused to let Annette clean
or straighten anything on it. Yet he could not manage to do it himself.
A breakthrough of sorts happened when a geriatric psychiatrist gave a
talk at Bright Ridge about dementia and Alzheimer's. Annette took Bill
to the discussion, and he agreed to make an appointment to see the psychiatrist. There was a six-month wait to see the doctor—not unusual for
a geriatric specialty practice. But during that time, Bill's paranoia
advanced. He would leave the apartment and sit in a darkened, empty
common room at Bright Ridge, or he would go down to the garage and
sit by their car.

"His paranoia was getting much worse," Annette says. "He didn't
want to go to the dining room to eat. I could see that it was because he
couldn't keep up with the conversation. He didn't want to have to talk
with anybody. He wasn't happy that I was active in volunteer work,
either. I would come home and he would be sitting in a chair. I had left
out a lunch for him at one point, but he wouldn't eat it because I wasn't
there to give it to him."

The geriatric psychiatrist diagnosed Bill as having a slowly progressive loss of cognitive abilities, including significant short-term memory
loss. After a series of tests, the doctor found that Bill could not handle
finances, and had lost some decision-making abilities. The psychiatrist
wrote a letter to Annette and Bill: "After reviewing available information, as well as the results of various tests and follow-up visits, I believe
that he suffers from significant dementia. In my opinion, the most likely
diagnosis is Alzheimer's disease, mild to moderate at this stage."

The doctor also found that Bill "has elements of significant depression" and prescribed an antidepressant. And he leveled with Annette: It
is clear, he said, that Bill should be in a supervised care setting, and his
dependency on caregivers will increase as time goes by. Newly married,
Annette was torn. They had so much in common, and he still had

moments of clarity. But she was also struggling with her own encroaching loss of mobility, relying more on a cane and a wheeled cart to maintain her balance. The social worker and staff at Bright Ridge were clearly worried. "One of the nurses who was working here came up to see us in the apartment and told us that we were going to find we couldn't stay together. He couldn't take care of me, and I couldn't take care of him. He had no response."

By this time, Annette thought they were right to be worried. Bill was becoming verbally abusive. "Here is one example," she says. "He had a big easy chair and he would open his mail. He would look at it and throw it on the floor all around his chair. I would go in and try to straighten up the room a little, and he would just get furious. He wouldn't want me to touch anything." Annette's children worried that his abuse would become physical, that one hard shove would send their increasingly fragile mother to the hospital with a broken hip, or worse. Bill began writing checks—one to a man he met at a grocery store who turned out to be running a tax-avoidance scam, one for someone representing an investment company who called frequently urging him to invest in land on the West Coast. "It was things like that that I just couldn't control," Annette says. She hired an organizer to bring some order to his desk, but the next day he began tearing out file folders and tossing them onto the floor.

Reluctantly, Annette's son arranged for a lawyer to work with her and with Bill's family to dissolve the marriage and to move him into the assisted living wing of Bright Ridge. The couple separated, and Annette extended an invitation to Bill to visit her every Sunday to read the newspaper and watch the news shows on television together. But the proximity didn't work. "I'd find him outside my door, crying," Annette says. "And he was spying on me. One day some friends of mine asked me to go to dinner with them in the dining room. On the second floor, looking down, there was Bill standing there watching us."

As Bill's dementia deepened, his children decided to move him west. His daughter helped him pack his belongings and moved him in with her, with home health aides to help with showers and a nearby doctor to supervise his medications. Annette gave him a cell phone so they could stay in touch, but he can no longer work it, so she calls him. He fades in and out, she says. "Sometimes, he'll talk and it is amazing. I'll talk about places where I have been to eat and he'll remember how to get there, what's on the menu. But that is happening less and less."

Annette had joined a support group at Bright Ridge for spouses when she was struggling with Bill's decline, but acknowledges that she was "in an upset mood when Bill left, because we'd been having a good time. It was fun to have him around. Until things fell apart."

Staff members feel their pain, certainly. Charles, an Alzheimer care coordinator at a nursing home in central Massachusetts, says, "It's not so easy to see a family coming in and leaving their family member with you and saying, 'You can take care of them.' It is so hard. A lot of them come in tears. You really have to put yourself in their shoes. Once they are used to it, you really help to make them feel that the decision to place their family member in your hands was the right one. You give them that assurance, and that exhibits itself because the next time they come, they see their family member happy, dressed nicely, groomed, looking as superbly as anybody else walking out on the street. Once they get to that stage, they can even forget they have that problem. At that point it really becomes a community, a coexistence."[10]

Beset by the downturn in the economy, many nursing homes are struggling. One of the nation's nursing home giants, Sunrise Senior Living, has been struggling with debt and downsizing, for example. Although Sunrise Senior Living reported that it posted a profit in the final quarter of 2009, it warned that it still has $440 million in debt. In the last two years, the company has been cutting its payroll and selling properties.[11]

A federal investigation conducted by the Department of Health and Human Services (HHS) found that in many nursing homes conditions could be better. Inspectors who examined 14,000 facilities per year found that in 2005, 2006, and 2007, more than 91 percent of nursing homes surveyed were cited for deficiencies, according to a report issued in September 2008 by Daniel Levinson, the inspector general of HHS. Although the percentage remained somewhat stable over those three years, it represents an increase over the last decade. By way of contrast, 81 percent of nursing homes were cited for deficiencies in 1998. Ninety-four percent of for-profit nursing homes were cited for deficiencies in 2007, according to the report, compared with 88 percent of nonprofits and 91 percent of homes run by government agencies. (The majority of nursing homes in the United States are owned by for-profit companies.) For-profit nursing homes also had a higher average number of deficiencies per home than other types of facilities. In 2007, for-profits averaged 7.6 deficiencies per home, not-for-profit homes averaged 5.7 deficiencies per home, and government homes averaged 6.3. The most common deficiency categories cited were quality of care, resident assessment, and quality of life. Perhaps most alarming, nearly 17 percent of nursing homes surveyed in 2007 were cited for deficiencies that could cause "immediate jeopardy" or "actual harm."

Charles acknowledges that the nursing home in Massachusetts has been affected by budget cuts, but he says the institution is working with the Service Employees International Union to identify savings without cutting programs. "We need to make sure that financial issues never get out of control," he said in an interview. "We are working in collaboration with the union and what they're trying to do is locate the problems that the industry is currently facing. We are not an exception; many institutions are facing the same problems. [The union] is trying to come up with solutions. We realize that there is a need for culture change to make sure that our residents, despite the problems, feel safe and comfortable as much as possible. And also that they're receiving the same care. There is a lot that needs to be done in the long term."

Violent behavior exhibited by a loved one, the unmitigated anger of a sudden inner mental storm, can also prompt a family to seek placement. Such a storm can erupt any time, during the most mundane errands—as it did for one family I saw. While a passenger in a car driven by his daughter, Mr. Tarlan (not his actual name) shouted at her, "You murdered twenty-five thousand children!" His daughter turned to him and saw him slowly shake his head as the storm gained strength. He blurted out at her, "I thought you were a lady of some comport."

For Mr. Tarlan, the commonly held view that Alzheimer's disease is primarily a memory problem seems far off the mark. Instead, the disease has introduced a Mr. Hyde into the otherwise healthy body of a Dr. Jekyll. Mr. Tarlan completely transformed himself when he became angry. Between episodes he was congenial, even witty, and able to dance around the surprising gaps in his knowledge. He could say what year it was or the name of the president, and his knowledge gaps would only surface when he was asked the questions directly—not something that usually happened in social settings. Mr. Tarlan could quite skillfully cover up these glaring information holes, but when some deep wellspring of anger rose up there was no way to cap it, and often the anger did not even have any apparent trigger. The random, unexpected nature of these outbursts made it all the more difficult. The disease was eating into a brain control center for anger.

If Mr. Tarlan had been in a nursing home, his behavior might have prompted the staff to reach for one of their most potent weapons—antipsychotic drugs. New drugs in this category are rolling out frequently, usually with an indication for the psychotic behavior observed with schizophrenia. According to the Centers for Medicare and Medicaid Services, 30 percent of nursing home residents are on antipsychotic medication, even though the vast majority do not have a primary psychosis. Instead, these drugs are being used for the behavioral symptoms of Alzheimer's disease. This surging use of these powerful drugs is occurring despite a "black box" warning label from the Food and Drug Administration (FDA) that these drugs increase the risk of death in demented elderly. In Britain, a recommendation against using two antipsychotics—olanzapine and risperidone—was issued by the Committee for the Safety of Medicines in 2004 due to an increased risk of stroke. These drugs can be viewed as sledge hammers that slam a broad swath of brain circuitry without specificity for any particular disease state. The often limitless manner in which the brain generates thoughts and ideas slows down as if encased in molasses. In general, these drugs work on neurochemical systems in the brain that control our mental states and are closely tied to the dopamine and serotonin pathways.

The earliest of these drugs was clozapine, but a side effect that wiped out certain blood cells prompted a search for similar acting drugs without such negative effects. In the 1990s, olanzapine, risperidone, and quetiapine were introduced, and in the 2000s ziprasidone, aripiprazole, and paliperidone followed. The newer drugs are called "atypical" because they were touted to have fewer side effects, in contrast to the older typical antipsychotics, such as the phenothiazines. However, it has become clear that the "atypicals" also can have significant side effects and may not be preferred over the older typical antipsychotics. Individuals taking these medications may actually have an increased tendency toward falls, somnolence, and abnormal gait. The large number of different antipsychotics available has led to some physicians branding themselves as psycho-neuro-pharmacologists. They specialize in designing—usually by trial and error—the optimal cocktail of drugs for the individual.

Possible long-term side effects of all antipsychotics include involuntary repetitive movements (tardive dyskinesia) that can persist even after the drug is withdrawn. Such movements often include grimacing, tongue protrusion, lip smacking, puckering and pursing of the lips, rapid eye blinking, or jerking-like movements of the limbs or fingers. People with these movements may not be fully aware of them and cannot control them. A related involuntary movement disorder is akathisia, or restlessness. Patients with this disorder cannot sit still and report feeling uncomfortable and tormented; they are up and down when interviewed by the doctor.

Although hard to sort out from the disease process itself, all antipsychotics may alter sleep patterns and induce fatigue and weakness. According to the safety inserts, these drugs also can reduce bone mineral density and lead to osteoporosis, weight gain, insulin resistance, hyperglycemia (or high levels of blood sugar), and diabetes. Some of the side effects due to use of antipsychotics are caused by an elevation of the hormone prolactin, which, along with another hormone, called oxytocin, is responsible for the interval immediately after orgasm when males cannot achieve an erection but feel a sense of gratification. High levels of prolactin may contribute to impotence and loss of sex drive.

In 2005, Medicaid spent $5.4 billion on atypical antipsychotic medications. This expense is greater than the price tag on any other class of drugs, including antibiotics for infections or antihypertensives for high blood pressure. The initial interest and popularity of these drugs coincided with the signing in 1987 of a federal law called the Nursing Home Reform Act that tightened the regulations over the use of physical and even chemical restraints such as typical antipsychotics in nursing homes. While the law did not prohibit the use of restraints entirely, it did set up strict guidelines and parameters that must be met before the use of restraints are considered appropriate.

In a retrospective conducted by Becky Briesacher at the University Massachusetts Medical School, 2.5 million Medicare beneficiaries in nursing homes during 2000–2001 were assessed for antipsychotic use and adherence to nursing home prescribing guidelines.[12] In addition to treatment for schizophrenia, antipsychotics may also be prescribed for delirium or dementia, but only if psychotic features or dangerous behaviors are also present. In the case of dementia, a behavioral assessment must show evidence of verbal or physical aggression, or delusions or hallucinations. In fact, these drugs have been used for wandering, restlessness, unsociability, uncooperativeness, and indifference to surroundings. And the presence of hallucinations, even when nondisturbing to the patient, is a highly questionable indication. Federal guidelines stipulate maximum daily doses for all antipsychotics and preclude the use of concurrent antipsychotics. Exceptions to these rules require documentation in the resident's record. If residents receive inappropriate antipsychotics without proper documentation, nursing homes may be cited by the government for deficient care and incur fines and sanctions.

According to the Briesacher's report, "Approximately 693,000, or 27.6 percent, of all Medicare beneficiaries in nursing homes received at least one prescription for antipsychotics during the study period. Less than half (41.8 percent) of treated residents received antipsychotic therapy in accordance with prescribing guidelines. One (23.4 percent) in four patients had no appropriate indication, 17.2 percent had daily doses exceeding recommended levels, and 17.6 percent had both inappropriate indications and high dosing. Patients receiving antipsychotic therapy within guidelines were no more likely to achieve stability or improvement in behavioral symptoms than were those taking antipsychotics outside the guidelines." The last finding is perhaps the most disturbing: even when antipsychotics are used, they did not reduce the targeted behaviors.

Another facet of this widespread use of drugs outside their intended purpose—atypical antipsychotics are only approved by the FDA for patients with schizophrenia or bipolar disorder, which causes manic periods of high energy and, then, deep depression—is that many of the drug recipients are Alzheimer patients who are unable to refuse the medication.[13] If family members object to the use these medications, the staff often threaten to discharge these patients because their behavior poses a danger to themselves or others. Nursing homes turn to drugs in part because it is a cheaper method of restraint than hiring more staff. (And, to be sure, the growing Alzheimer burden makes it more and more difficult to find staff.) They also turn to drugs because behavior issues are viewed as a medical problem in need of a medical solution—and the natural tendency of the medical community is to prescribe drugs. However, a nonmedical approach, while by no means a panacea, can sometimes be more effective: massages, aromatherapy, playing music that holds memories, and engaging patients in activities can prove to be soothing according to many personal accounts.

THE ALZHEIMER EPIDEMIC IS COMING AT A TIME WHEN THE HEALTHCARE SYSTEM IS IN PERIL

From doctors to patients to administrators to politicians, few would give our healthcare system good marks. The failures inherent in the system affect not only our health but the economic vitality of many large corporations. US healthcare expenditures exceeded $2 trillion in 2006—equal to $7,000 per person and estimated to be $2.4 trillion in 2008. Health is the most expensive sector of our economy, by far, four times larger than national defense. Sixteen percent of the gross domestic product was allocated to healthcare in 2006—double the 8.8 percent of twenty-five years earlier, according to a 2007 report by the Organization for Economic Co-operation and Development.[14] At present growth rates, US expenditures on healthcare will reach $4 trillion and 20 percent of the gross domestic product by 2015.[15] A typical US worker pays $3,000 for family coverage, a 150 percent increase since the year 2000, a soaring rise during a period when healthcare inflation was 25 percent. The premiums paid by employers average $11,500 for family coverage, a figure that exceeds the annual wages for a minimum wage worker.[16]

The challenges we face in securing affordable healthcare for elders are closely linked to the Medicare program. Medicare accounts for about 20 percent of our health spending, and its payment rules are widely adopted by private insurers in setting their own policies for coverage and reimbursement of health services. Although Medicare provides essentially universal coverage to people over age sixty-five, those covered incur mounting out-of-pocket costs. Medicare reimbursements that do not cover the physician's costs have caused some doctors to close their practices to new Medicare clients, which impedes patient access to specialists. Once she is in a nursing home, care for a Medicare patient is limited. According to the Centers for Medicare and Medicaid Services, the average time spent in caring for a patient in nursing homes is thirty minutes from a registered nurse, forty-eight minutes from a licensed practical nurse, and two hours and eighteen minutes from an aide. As baby boomers begin to enroll in Medicare starting in 2011, these problems will escalate and, according to the Medicare trustees, assets in the Part A trust fund will be exhausted in 2019.[17]

Suggestions for repair of the system are coming from all directions across the political spectrum: from economists, union members, physicians, and from examples of what appears to work in other countries. What surfaces to the public is a big-hammer approach that appears to mandate sweeping changes in coverage. But the debaters fail to recognize that health is not a monolithic entity. It actually encompasses a multitude of issues, which differ according to a patient's medical condition, age, geographic proximity to medical services, and cultural and economic status. The lack of uniformity of healthcare needs is reflected in the distribution of expenditures. The most costly 1 percent of individuals accounts for 20 to 30 percent of total expenditures. The most costly 5 percent of individuals accounts for 50 percent of total expenditures, and the most costly 20 percent of people accounts for 80 percent of total expenditures. On the other side of the curve, the least costly 50 percent accounts for only 3 percent of total expenditures, and 15 percent of the general population incurs no medical expenses during the year.[18]

The distribution of expenditures is heavily skewed toward the elderly, whose costs far exceed those of the average individual. The numbers of people who fall into this category has grown rapidly—life expectancy has increased by ten years since 1950, the Medicare population has quintupled since 1965, and patients with costly chronic diseases are living longer. These patients are expected to create a strain on families as hospital stays shorten and homecare technology advances. In a 2008 study titled "Assuring Healthy Caregivers," the Centers for Disease Control and Prevention (CDC) in Atlanta predicted that the number of family caregivers will grow by eighty-five percent from 2000 to 2050. "A substantial portion of supportive care services rendered today is provided outside of the formal medical care system, having been transferred to the community where families now serve as primary caregivers in the home," the study, says. Between 2000 and 2030, the number of people sixty-five and older will rise 101 percent—or 2.3 percent each year.[19]

"Unfortunately," the CDC study says, "over that same thirty-year period, the number of family members who are available to provide care for these older adults is expected to increase by only 25 percent, at a rate of 0.8 percent per year." The CDC, citing data from the National Alliance for Caregiving and the AARP, found that, as of 2004, caregivers were already present in one out of every five households in the United States. The majority—83 percent—were unpaid family members, friends, or neighbors. The remaining 17 percent were paid professionals obtained through a service. One-quarter of all caregivers of people age fifty or older are providing help to someone with cognitive impairment, memory problems, or Alzheimer's disease, the CDC report found.

So it is no surprise that the repair of the US healthcare system, broadly defined as healthcare reform, has dominated political discussions. Even the more esoteric facets of the debate, such as "individual mandates"—a policy that would require individuals to purchase health insurance—emerged in a candidates' debate and shows a deepening concern about our sputtering system of care and the aging of the baby boom generation.

Hillary Clinton, secretary of state in the Obama administration, fulfilled another role during her husband's first term in office: She oversaw an effort to reform the healthcare system that ultimately foundered. While the bill she and her team of advisers produced was sweeping in scope, at more than 1,300 pages, the process she engendered was criticized as opaque. Critics in Congress said they felt shut out. The infamous "Harry and Louise" ad campaign mounted by the insurance industry stoked fears of a giant bureaucracy that would forever kill the notion of choice.

In the 2008 presidential campaign, however, Harry and Louise returned, now middle-aged and worried about the rising cost of healthcare—and perhaps their own mortality.

Clinton shared some insights into the issues that healthcare analysts should tackle next. Chronic diseases—and prevention—must be addressed, she said in an e-mail interview.[20] "Our healthcare system must do more to address chronic diseases, which account for the vast majority of costs. We need to realign the incentives in our system to emphasize prevention and avoid the costly complications associated with diseases like diabetes, where an amputation costs far more than nutrition counseling or diabetes management," she said.

As the system is changed, Clinton said, gaps in knowledge must be addressed, too. "Certain chronic diseases, like Alzheimer's, are still largely a mystery to us. We don't know much about their causes, or what preventive measures might be taken to reduce their impact. We don't have cost-effective early detection methods, and need to make gains in effective treatment," she said. Clinton looked ahead to how any potential healthcare reform plan should attempt to address diseases such as Alzheimer's. "Health reform also must look at the gaps in our understanding of chronic disease and expand research efforts to help find the causes, effective screening tools, best treatments, and eventual cures for diseases like Alzheimer's," she said. "At the same time, we need to raise awareness of Alzheimer's and support the families and caregivers of those living with this disease, including expansion of home and community-based care and services."

Before his death in August 2009, US Senator Edward M. Kennedy, whose family was touched by long-term illness even before his own diagnosis of brain cancer, vowed to make healthcare reform the cause of his life. As chair of the powerful Senate Committee on Health, Education, Labor, and Pensions, he established three working groups and asked them to focus on critical issues. The first, under Senator Tom Harkin, an Iowa Democrat, will investigate the areas of prevention and public health. Senator Barbara Mikulski, a Maryland Democrat, will lead a group on improvements in quality, and a third group will focus on insurance.

Kennedy noted that, as a senator, he had high-quality health insurance and could consult with the best specialists in the country after his cancer diagnosis in May 2008. But his experience as a parent of children who needed medical treatment also made a deep impression on him. In his book *America Back on Track*, he identifies healthcare as one of the seven major challenges facing society and calls for a program that assures Medicare for all.[21]

Businesses shaken by the faltering economy are laying off employees, leaving them with few options for affordable healthcare after the interim insurance policy provided under COBRA runs out—unless they can find new jobs quickly or qualify for Medicare. (COBRA, an abbreviation of the Consolidated Omnibus Budget Reconciliation Act, allows workers who lose health benefits to continue their group health benefits from their former job for a limited time, although premium payments increase.)[22] While free markets work well for goods such as cars and computers, Kennedy believes, medical services and medical outcomes are different.

Tom Daschle, whose nomination for secretary of Health and Human Services ultimately foundered, was not only a longtime friend of Kennedy's, but shares his passion for retooling healthcare. At his confirmation hearing in January 2009, Daschle staked out his ground quickly. "The flaws in our health system are pervasive and corrosive," he told the Senate Committee on Health, Education, Labor, and Pensions. "They threaten our health and economic security."[23]

Daschle noted the failed effort at health reform in 1994, during the Clinton administration, and assessed the costs. In essence, he said, time is ticking away, and he expressed a fear that harsh economic realities and gaps in care can negate the most cutting-edge scientific research. "While our investments in research and pioneering work by our scientists lead innovation," he told the panel, too often patients don't actually get our best. In 1994, we had thirty-seven million Americans who were uninsured. Today that number is forty-six million. In 1987, one dollar out of fifteen went toward healthcare for the average family. Today, it's one out of six."

Like many people, he finds value in a system that would pay doctors for comprehensive preventive care. "Any healthcare reform plan must make sure that every American has preventive care that prevents disease and disability. Coverage after you get sick should be a second line of defense. Today it's often the first line," he testified. "In addition to being sound medicine, this is sound fiscal policy. Studies have shown that every dollar spent on prevention could actually net a return of $5.60 in healthcare costs, totaling upwards of $16 billion annually within five years."

The Obama administration's secretary of Health and Human Services, Kathleen Sebelius, told Senators at her confirmation hearing in April 2009 that her experience as a governor showed her how healthcare reform could work at a statewide level. Kansas, she said, has lessons for the nation. "I was asked by my predecessor, Republican Governor Bill Graves, to lead the team to design and implement the Children's Health Insurance Program [CHIP]," Sebelius testified on April 2, 2009, before the Senate Finance Committee. "Our separate insurance initiative called Health Wave is modeled on the state employee program. Its enrollment started at 15,000 in the first year; today, it covers over 51,000 children. And the Legislature just voted to support my recommendation that our CHIP program be expanded," Sebelius said.

She listed her accomplishments in Kansas that might be relevant to any national program. "I have also worked to make lifesaving medications affordable. I established counseling programs to help seniors navigate the complicated Medicare prescription drug benefit plan," she said. "When seniors started falling through the cracks of the new drug program, I directed the state to pay their prescription costs to Kansas pharmacies to prevent the loss of coverage. During this period, we filled 45,000 prescriptions for Medicare-eligible seniors," she said.[24]

Senator Max Baucus, a Democrat from Montana and chairman of the Senate Finance Committee, held his own healthcare summit in June 2008. His voluminous white paper, "Reforming America's Health Care System: A Call to Action,"[25] issued in November 2008, won praise from Kennedy, who gave it his imprimatur and signaled a bipartisan effort in a statement: "I look forward to working with Senator Baucus, our colleagues in Congress on both sides of the aisle, and the Obama administration to see that we at last achieve the goal of quality, affordable healthcare for all Americans. Senator Baucus's white paper brings us closer to that goal."[26]

Baucus found that healthcare concerns are closely linked to the economic anxiety engulfing the nation, and that 62 percent of voters in the 2008 presidential elections had healthcare reform on their minds as they pulled the lever. "This moment in history is not unlike that faced by President Franklin D. Roosevelt and the New Deal generation as they sought a path out of the Great Depression," he wrote. "Now, as then, solving America's economic challenges will require a multifaceted response. Reforming the nation's healthcare system will be an essential part of shoring up the nation's long-term economic health."

Baucus proposes the creation of a nationwide insurance pool called the Health Insurance Exchange. The exchange would allow those who had health insurance to keep their plan, but would guarantee affordable coverage for the uninsured by providing a marketplace where consumers could compare plans and buy what they wanted. Insurers who offered coverage through the exchange would have to meet requirements established by a new Independent Health Coverage Council. The plan would shore up employer-based health insurance. Employers who did not offer healthcare would have to contribute to a fund to help cover the uninsured. During the period it took to create and fund the exchange, the Baucus plan would extend Medicare to Americans beginning at age fifty-five. The plan would also provide everyone living below the poverty level with access to Medicaid. Baucus acknowledges that federal funds would be needed to start the exchange, but perhaps optimistically, he believes that the program would be self-sustaining within a few years.

The pharmaceutical industry is busy predicting the impact of the aging baby-boom generation and what it means for Alzheimer's drugs. In 2007, Robert Essner, then chief executive of the drug company Wyeth, told *New York Times* reporter Stephanie Saul that Alzheimer's may be one of the biggest healthcare and political issues of his generation.[27] (Essner was then fifty-nine, an age that put him squarely in the baby boom.) He called on the National Institutes of Health to double its annual funding of Alzheimer's research (in 2007, that amounted to $643 million) and committed three hundred fifty Wyeth scientists to work exclusively on Alzheimer's disease. Essner had presumably done the math. A successful drug could cost patients up to $20,000 a year, and the number of cases could grow to 13.2 million by 2050, according to National Institute on Aging estimates.

Brian Rosman, research director of Health Care for All, a nonprofit agency in Massachusetts dedicated to working on affordable healthcare, puts it another way: the healthcare system is completely upside down. Doctors and hospitals are paid on a piecework basis, by procedure or by office visit. "There is no coordination," he said in a telephone interview, "and no one is paid to look after the patient as a whole. This fragmented system rewards high-intensity services, and it rewards specialty care over primary care. No one gets paid for sitting down with a patient and talking with them about risk factors and healthy nutrition and things like that."[28]

Rosman would like to see "a complete reversal of how the payment structure works, with a focus on the 'medical home.' It's not an ideal name, because people think it refers to a physical place. Instead, it's more a way of organizing care that puts the patient at the center and has a team of people who are paid to keep the patient healthy."

A Massachusetts physician who does work on healthcare policy boils the problem down to its essence: direct patient care. "We need to get much more involved in getting the patient's perspective in terms of how empowered he or she is." This physician suggests rewarding healthcare providers on the basis of improvement. "It doesn't have to be that the patient is getting better, because obviously in dementia the patient does not necessarily get better. However, one can certainly reward on the basis of a whole other set of issues that are not rewarded today. An outcome might be based on patient or family satisfaction."[29]

In an assessment of the staggering costs of Alzheimer's done in 2006, the Alzheimer's Association predicted that annual Medicare and Medicaid costs of treating beneficiaries with Alzheimer's disease will increase 65 percent by 2011. The cost to American business: an estimated $61 billion a year—$24.6 billion to cover healthcare and $36.5 billion for caregiver absenteeism and loss of production.[30] The authors of the study decry budget cuts proposed by the Bush administration that reduced funding for Alzheimer's research by approximately $4 million and placed additional financial restrictions on who could qualify for Medicaid nursing home coverage.

"The human and economic impact of Alzheimer's disease—on individuals robbed of memory and ability to function independently, on families overwhelmed by the emotional, financial, and physical burdens of care, and on healthcare programs that will not be able to sustain the growing numbers of people with the disease—provide compelling reasons for accelerating progress toward reaching our goal of a world without Alzheimer's. However, in the midst of a growing budget deficit, the federal government has decreased its commitment to biomedical research, and funding for programs that support individuals with Alzheimer's disease and their caregivers is in jeopardy," the report says.

The authors issue a dire warning, grounded in data on funding trends and demographics: "If this trend continues, Alzheimer's will strap our country with a huge burden of elderly disability and devastate our economy and healthcare system. The economic and demographic impact of Alzheimer's disease, brought on by the aging of the baby boomers, is a direct threat to the retirement security of millions of American families and to the fiscal security of the entire nation."

Although Medicare does not cover long-term care, and Medicaid is available only after a lifetime of savings has been depleted, costs associated with Alzheimer's could prove overwhelming, the Alzheimer's Association report finds. Medicare spending for people with Alzheimer's is expected to soar to $189 billion by 2015—before most baby boomers are at an age where their risk for the disease would be expected to rise.

Is there a potential solution? The Alzheimer's Association calls on Congress to add a Medicare chronic care benefit, citing a potential for enormous savings in hospital stays. It recommends including payments for a physician or other professional to coordinate patient care and help caregivers navigate the system, and recommends reimbursing physicians who counsel weary family caregivers outside of office visits. ("Currently, Medicare will not reimburse for this service," the report notes, "diminishing the quality of communication between the caregiver and the physician, which can be detrimental to patient safety as well as caregiver confidence and well-being.")

The Alzheimer's Association study also recommends extending Medicare to patients under sixty-five who are diagnosed with early onset Alzheimer's. The report cites data which show that almost one-third of people aged fifty-five to sixty-four with cognitive impairment do not have health insurance. "With or without health insurance, many people with early onset dementia and their families are likely to face very high out-of-pocket expenditures for long-term care or be forced to forgo medical care."

Economist Robert Kuttner argues that a comprehensive national system is better positioned to match resources with needs. Writing a "second opinion" in the New England Journal of Medicine, Kuttner pronounces healthcare a "market-based failure."[31] While medical inflation has been tied to the aging population, he believes instead that "the extreme failure of the United States to contain medical costs results primarily from our unique, pervasive commercialization." Kuttner, cofounder of the liberal journal American Prospect and a senior fellow at Demos, a public policy research and advocacy organization with offices in New York City, Washington, DC, and Boston, continues this thread: "The dominance of for-profit insurance and pharmaceutical companies, a new wave of investor-owned specialty hospitals, and profit-maximizing behavior even by nonprofit players raise costs and distort resource allocation," he writes. Kuttner contends that the healthcare system is dominated by business and commercial interests that do not put patients first. "Profits, billing, marketing, and the gratuitous costs of private bureaucracies siphon off $400 billion to $500 billion of the $2.1 trillion spent, but the more serious and less appreciated syndrome is the set of perverse incentives produced by commercial dominance of the system."

Eric J. Hall, president and CEO of the Alzheimer's Foundation of America, said policymakers are starting to look at cognitive issues in a different light. "I have to say that I don't believe federal officials give much credence to cognitive issues or mental capacity in this regard, unless it directly impinges upon ADLs [activities of daily living]. It's not CMS's [the federal Centers for Medicare and Medicaid Services] fault, however," he says in a telephone interview.[32] "At the time CMS was created, we didn't have people living into their eighties and nineties. The program as it was established was tremendously effective, and I respect the model. I think now, given the environment and given the aging population and given the growth of this and other related disorders, it is our hope that policymakers will enable CMS to broaden its interpretation of the well-being of a person beyond just the physical."

While he stresses that he would love to see a cure, he doubts that a magical silver bullet is on the near horizon. In the absence of a cure, Hall says, prevention and care become top priorities. Alzheimer's disease is more likely to be treated with a mixture of treatments that will offset the symptoms for a longer period of time, he believes. Because of this likely progression, Hall sees a need to "speak clearly and definitively" about screening and early diagnosis. "We need to get the whole country to be more proactive about memory problems and perhaps doctors begin asking, 'How has your memory been?'"

NOTES

1. Alzheimer's Association, "2009 Alzheimer's Disease Facts and Figures," http://www.alz.org/alzheimers_disease_facts_figures.asp.

2. US Census Bureau data available at http://www.census.gov/.

3. Alzheimer's Association, "2009 Alzheimer's Disease Facts."

4. Lucette Lagnado, "Nursing Homes Struggle to Kick Drug Habit," *Wall Street Journal*, December 20, 2007, p.1.

5. Information on the Framingham Heart Study can be found at http://www.framinghamheartstudy.org/.

6. "I Can't Remember," *BusinessWeek*, September 2003.

7. Alice Munro, *Away from Her / The Bear Came over the Mountain* (New York: Vintage, 2007).

8. Jan Thorgaard (pseudonym), telephone interview with Ellen Clegg, February 2009.

9. Annette Edmonds (pseudonym), telephone interview with Ellen Clegg, February 2009.

10. Interview by Michele Cerulli, December 2008.

11. Jeff Clabaugh, "Sunrise Posts Profit, Faces Default," *Washington Business Journal*, February 25, 2010, http://washington.bizjournals.com/washington/stories/2010/02/22/daily56.html.

12. Becky Briesacher et al., "The Quality of Antipsychotic Drug Prescribing in Nursing Homes," *Archives of Internal Medicine* 165, no. 11 (June 13, 2005): 1280–85.

13. "Randomized Controlled Trial of the Effect on Quality of Life of Second- vs. First-Generation Antipsychotic Drugs in Schizophrenia: Cost Utility of the Latest Antipsychotic Drugs in Schizophrenia Study," (CUtLASS 1), *Archives of General Psychiatry* 63, no. 10:1079–87.

14. Organization for Economic Cooperation and Development, OECD Health Data 2007, http://www.oecd.org/health/healthdata.

15. C. Borger et al., "Health Spending Projections through 2015: Changes on the Horizon," *Health Affairs* Web exclusive 25 (2006): W61–W73.

16. Henry J. Kaiser Family Foundation, "Medicare Fact Sheet: Medicare at a Glance" (Menlo Park, CA: Henry J. Kaiser Family Foundation, February 2007), publication no. 1066–10.

17. Social Security and Medicare Boards of Trustees, "Status of the Social Security and Medicare Programs: A Summary of the 2008 Annual Reports," March 25, 2008, http://www.ssa.gov/OACT/TRSUM/trsummary.html (accessed April 10, 2008).

18. M. L. Beck and A. C. Monheit, "The Concentration of Health Expenditures, Revisited," *Health Affairs* 20 (2001): 9–18; Medicare Payment Advisory Commission, Reports to the Congress, Washington, DC, June 2004.

19. Centers for Disease Control and Prevention and the Kimberly-Clark Corporation, "Assuring Healthy Caregivers," http://www.cdc.gov/aging/.

20. Hillary Clinton, e-mail interview with Ellen Clegg, December 2008.

21. Senator Edward M. Kennedy, *America Back on Track* (New York: Penguin, 2007).

22. US Department of Labor, http://www.dol.gov/dol/topic/health-plans/cobra.htm (accessed July 8, 2009).

23. Senator Tom Daschle's testimony, transcribed by CQ Transcription, January 8, 2009, http://www.nytimes.com/2009/01/08/us/politics/08text-daschle.html.

24. Transcript, Senate Finance Committee, April 2, 2009, finance.senate.gov/hearings/testimony/2009test/040209kstest.pdf (accessed July 8, 2009).

25. Senator Max Baucus, "A Call to Action," http://finance.senate.gov/healthreform2009/home.html.

26. Senator Kennedy's statement from http://finance.senate.gov/healthreform2009/support.html.

27. Stephanie Saul, "Taking on Alzheimer's," *New York Times*, June 10, 2007, http://www.nytimes.com/2007/06/10/business/yourmoney/10alz.html.

28. Brian Rosman, telephone interview with Ellen Clegg, January 2009.

29. Telephone interview with Ellen Clegg, January 2009.

30. Alzheimer's Association, "2006 National Public Policy Program to Conquer Alzheimer's Disease," http://www.alz.org/advocacy/2006program/1.asp.

31. "Market-Based Failure—A Second Opinion on US Health Care Costs," *New England Journal of Medicine* 358, no. 6 (February 7, 2008).

32. Eric Hall, telephone interview with Ellen Clegg, February 2009.

6

A DANCE WITH TWO PARTNERS

The Marketplace and the Regulators

THE SYSTEM STYMIES PHYSICIAN CREATIVITY

> The individual physician has virtually no opportunity to offer a different bundle of services for a different price. As a result, very little entrepreneurship is possible.
>
> —JOHN C. GOODMAN, PRESIDENT OF THE
> NATIONAL CENTER FOR POLICY ANALYSIS

The very market forces that have fostered large bureaucracies have also stymied creativity within the medical community. Massive third-party payer groups not only impose prices and contracts but also gobble up a giant share of US healthcare expenditures. Size seems to work against efficiency. In contrast to Medicare, which spends 3 percent of its funds on administrative overhead and is able to deliver fairly prompt electronic payment, the complex and protracted payment systems of private insurance carriers spend 12 to 15 percent of their income on administrative overhead and profits. In 2005, the costs for health insurance administration and profits as a percentage of all US healthcare expenditures were 13 percent of the $2 trillion spent and were a higher expenditure than physician income, nursing home care, or medications. The gross income of physicians has actually fallen from 19 percent to 16 percent of total healthcare costs while time spent on patient care has risen from 47.2 hours to 50.1 hours weekly.[1]

Simple technologies such as the telephone and e-mail, used by most professionals, are not reimbursed by Medicare/BlueCross. Doctors are paid by Medicare/BlueCross for 7,500 specific tasks, none of which include the telephone or e-mail. As John C. Goodman of the National Center for Policy Analysis cogently points out, physicians who are already stretched to the maximum have little incentive to attract more patients by implementing patient-pleasing modifications. A healthcare system able to incorporate the leading-edge trends of market forces can operate without necessarily leaving the underserved behind, however.

In contrast to the stifling atmosphere of third-party payment systems, market-driven systems are thriving in certain sectors. Lasik surgery on the eye to correct nearsightedness and out-of-pocket payments for prescription drugs at sites like Rx.com are able to compete on price and quality. According to Goodman, while technological innovation has occurred in Lasik surgery, the price has dropped 30 percent over the past ten years. The business of cosmetic surgery, not covered by private insurance, is booming among the well-to-do. Walk-in clinics in shopping malls and drugstores have short wait times, electronic records are widely used, and service is comparable to traditional primary care at half the cost.

These innovative settings are beginning to change the face of the traditional medical care model. In contrast to traditional medical settings, prices are posted. Few hospitals list their charges, much less the accompanying professional fees and the out-of-pocket costs; instead, a bill, often replete with unpleasant surprises, arrives weeks or months later. And medical "tourism," a euphemistic term applied to US citizens who travel outside the country for medical care and surgical procedures at cut rates, is increasingly adopted to get affordable care. In the face of all these changes, Alzheimer's disease services, and particularly Alzheimer's disease prevention programs, are in sore need of innovation on the supply side.

Our knowledge of individual differences in a patient's disease risk and response to medications is expanding rapidly. But the by-product of this knowledge—personalized medicine—lags behind the times. In a recent issue of the *Harvard Business Review*, Mara Aspinall and Richard Hamermesh listed four barriers to the medical community shifting from what they call "trial-and-error" to personalized medicine. (If you want to see trial-and-error in action, watch a physician as he prescribes medication for treating Alzheimer's disease. Three of the four available drugs—galantamine [Razadyne, formerly known as Reminyl], rivastigmin [Exelon], and donepezil [Aricept]—all work similarly, but may differ in their tendencies to cause gastrointestinal side effects, such as nausea and vomiting. Typically, doctors try one of these drugs and if the patient encounters problems, it is on to the next.)

Throughout this book we have touched upon all of these barriers, but here they are in list form:

(1) The blockbuster model of drug marketing discourages development of therapies for smaller population segments. In the case of Alzheimer's disease, many important population segments exist such as those with familial Alzheimer's disease and the many disorders with obscure names related to Alzheimer's disease such as Lewy body dementia, frontotemporal dementia, and progressive supranuclear palsy, among others.

(2) The regulatory environment puts excessive weight on Phase Three clinical trials (those using human subjects) in a final throw of the dice, with hundreds of millions of dollars at stake. The odds of rolling the winning number and getting an effective drug are strongly stacked against the success of a new drug.

(3) The dysfunctional payment system is based on procedures and prescriptions, rather than early diagnosis and prevention.

(4) Physicians are slow to adopt change.

REGULATION: CAN'T LIVE WITH IT AND CAN'T LIVE WITHOUT IT

While Alzheimer's disease certainly takes its place among the major killer diseases, we have noted that, unlike the other common killers such as heart disease and cancer, no facet of Alzheimer's disease requires surgery. Instead, most of the physician-related skills and services needed to diagnose and treat Alzheimer's disease fall well within the realm of primary care. As a neurologist, I am well aware that some of my neurology colleagues will object to this viewpoint. Indeed, the diagnostic skills of a neurologist are preferable in order to distinguish among some of the more obscure dementias.

Unfortunately, few, if any, treatments for the non-Alzheimer dementias exist that require their precise identification, so one could argue that imprecise diagnosis carries few consequences. (A notable exception is in the arena of research where precise diagnosis of non-Alzheimer dementias has yielded numerous clinical and basic insights. One of the leading centers for recognizing the non-Alzheimer dementias is led by Bruce Miller at the University of California at San Francisco.) Diseases such as frontotemporal dementia and Lewy body dementia are among the many diseases that can masquerade as Alzheimer's disease. Fortunately, their incidence trails far behind that of Alzheimer's disease.

In most community-based settings, there are not enough neurologists available to see the rapidly growing number of Alzheimer patients. Even among neurologists, many limit their practice to avoid Alzheimer patients, preferring more lucrative diagnoses that involve sophisticated and technical procedures to perform. After the diagnosis of Alzheimer's disease is made, the medical decisions required to manage this diagnosis are few (the social decisions, on the other hand, are many), and during the long, downhill course of the disease, a primary-care physician is well suited to the task. As the disease progresses, patients may need strong tranquilizers to curb behavioral symptoms—one family asked for tranquilizers for a sibling with Alzheimer's who would scream out in frustration and try to strike people with her cane, and an elderly spouse sought sedation for her husband because he had begun to shove her. This is not so much an issue of physician expertise as it is a part of treatment that requires careful monitoring of dose and side effects. (And, unfortunately, chronic care settings frequently do a poor job.) Alzheimer's disease is progressive, and therefore, the dose or even the need for a medication may diminish with time.

A complicated picture is made even murkier because regulators have created a strong disincentive among physicians to see Alzheimer patients. In the arcane world of medical billing, the particular billing codes used by primary-care doctors have been progressively undercompensated in the US healthcare market. These billing codes favor procedures—for example, surgeries and tests. This fiscal incentive increases the number performed, reduces the number of undercompensated visits without a procedure, and drives up medical costs.[2]

Since 1992, payments for physicians' services through Medicare have utilized something called RVUs, or relative-value units. The value units are a uniform "currency" used to measure the physician's actual work, the cost of maintaining the practice, and the cost of liability insurance.[3]

An analysis of the growth in RVUs per Medicare beneficiary from 1992 to 2002 revealed that the largest drivers of growth were major procedures. While fields such as cardiology and gastroenterology are awash with procedures, all assigned to their big-ticket billing codes, the physician visit with an Alzheimer patient does not generally involve procedures. Unlike the treadmill test or a colonoscopy, the few tests that might be ordered for Alzheimer's disease—such as neuropsychological testing or a brain scan—are not performed by the physician who is managing the case and are usually only done once. Most of our impact on Alzheimer's disease lies in the area of prevention—not an intervention that requires a procedure.

Therefore, Medicare's administered pricing system needs to set prices that fully reflect the value that the medical market places on specific services provided by particular physicians. Prices are the same regardless of the skill of the physician or the outcome for the patient. This is the issue of cost effectiveness, which is anathema for some in healthcare where the belief that we should not spare any expense to improve health pervades. But that view is full of self-delusion because those who cannot afford healthcare do, in fact, go without it. Furthermore, the purveyors of healthcare products and pharmaceuticals have taken advantage of our willingness to pay regardless of the cost.

Market valuation is best measured by the demands of patients, particularly elders who rely most heavily on Medicare, and the successful medical outcomes that result from such services. Defining a successful medical outcome in Alzheimer's disease represents a radically different problem than a successful outcome from cardiac bypass surgery. Exactly how to price services has been a thorn for Medicare since its inception in 1965. At first, the program compensated physicians on the basis of their charges and allowed them to bill beneficiaries for the full amount above what Medicare paid for each service. In 1975, compensation remained linked to what physicians charged, but the annual increase in fees was capped by an economic index. Payments continued to rise, so from 1984 through 1991, the yearly change in fees was determined by legislation. In 1992, the payment system based on physicians' charges was replaced by a fee schedule and the debacle of top-down pricing emerged. Payment for individual services was based on measures of the relative resources used to provide them, with the reasonable intention of redistributing spending among various physician specialties more equitably. But the mechanism led to highly variable changes in payment rates, so Congress replaced it with a new mechanism—the sustainable growth rate (SGR)—starting in 1998.

Although innocently named, the sustainable growth rate is mired in complexity. It is a formula more appropriately pondered by the complex mind of a Steven J. Hawking than the legislators who devised it. The formula describes how Medicare payments can accommodate increases in the volume and complexity of physician services at a rate supported by growth in national income. Just in case anyone wants to take a peek at one iteration of the formula, to judge the complexity physicians are wrestling with, here it is:

Change in physicians' prices (**1.026**) × change in enrollment (**0.971**) × change in real GDP per capita (**1.022**) × changes in law or regulation (**0.990**) = 1.007

If increases in payments exceed the SGR, an automatic cut in fees is triggered. Not surprisingly, looming in the very near term is the dreaded fee cut. As is often the case with regulation, the element of human behavior is missing in the formula. The system did not have the desired effect on physicians; they did not moderate their practice patterns, and judgment day grew nearer. Because outlays for physicians grew faster than permitted by the SGR, a substantial fee reduction would automatically be imposed. When the fee cut for physicians was to go into effect, Congress deferred the cut, which could lead to an even larger cut in coming years. All parties are currently boxed in without any good options: SGR-calculated fee cuts are growing, as are the costs of a temporary fix. As recently summed up by Joseph Antos, referring to the SGR impasse, "That uncertainty can discourage long-term investments in health information technology and other equipment to make physician practices more efficient, and it can discourage physicians from expanding their Medicare patient load."[4] The relatively low reimbursement physicians see from Alzheimer patients and the likelihood of further decline places this patient segment on the chopping block as physicians attempt to sustain their practices.

PAYING HIGH PRICES FOR DRUGS WITH MODEST EFFECTS

For those who cannot afford to pay for medications because they have no insurance or are saddled with high co-pays from the insurance plans they do have, the financial sacrifice may outweigh the benefits of the medication. However, big pharmaceutical companies play upon the powerful attachments people feel to afflicted family members and the guilt they experience if any treatment, no matter how minimal the effects, is withheld. I have seen over and over again patients who struggle to pay for one of the Alzheimer drugs on the market even though the benefits are short term and very modest at best. An example is the case of donepezil, which goes by the commercial name of Aricept. In October 2006, the FDA approved donepezil for patients with severe Alzheimer's disease. The drug had previously been approved for mild to moderate dementia in 1996. The 2006 decision was based on two clinical trials submitted by the drug's sponsors, Eisai Inc. and Pfizer Inc. One study, in *Lancet*, the British medical journal, followed 248 patients with severe dementia in a Swedish nursing home for six months.[5] Patients were given tests to measure their cognitive ability, and even relatively small positive changes were touted as the result of effective treatment, even though these changes had minimal impact on a patient's function.

Of the patients who completed the trial, ninety-five were given donepezil and ninety-nine were given a useless placebo. The outcomes measured were grouped under a battery of tests called the "severe impairment battery" (SIB), which measures memory, language, orientation (knowing one's location in space and time), attention, motor skills, visuospatial construction (the ability to draw or copy shapes), recalling the names of people and objects, and social interaction. The investigators also used another outcome measure based on a widely used test called the Alzheimer Disease Cooperative Study of Activities of Daily Living Inventory for Severe Alzheimer's Disease (ADCS-ADL-severe). In this test, nineteen measures of basic activities—such as the ability to feed and bathe oneself—and complex abilities—such as opening water taps and switching on lights—were measured. Scores on this test range from 0 to 54.

After six months, the treated group improved their SIB by an average of 5.7 points and improved their ADCS-ADL-severe test scores by 1.7 points. In both cases, the improvement was statistically significant. But as we will see in a moment, statistical significance on a neuropsychological test does not translate very well into an improvement in one's quality of life. A second, unpublished study from Japan was cited in the report to the FDA.[6] In this study, 325 patients were given differing levels of donepezil treatment or placebo for six months. On the SIB scale, patients on the higher dose of 10 mg improved by 4.7 points, those on the lower dose of 5 mg improved by 2.5 points, and placebo-treated patients declined by 4.2 points. The group from Japan also tested patients with the Clinician's Interview-Based Impression of Change Plus Caregiver Input (CIBIC-Plus), which is a highly structured interview, that is, all patients are asked the same questions and their responses are scored. In this study no significant differences related to the treatment were detected.

When the FDA approval of the drug for severe Alzheimer's disease was announced, Russell Katz, the director of the FDA's Division of Neurological Products, issued this semiapologetic statement: "It's fair to say that these drugs aren't cures or miraculous treatments. The average response both on the cognitive and global functioning measures is relatively small, there is no denying that."[7]

By small changes, Katz means that the interviewer, whose scores inevitably have some degree of subjectivity, thought a nursing home patient receiving assistance with many activities of daily living performed better on some small fraction of those activities. No claim is made that the level of care got better for nursing home patients or that the costs of caring for the person came down. In fact, costs may have risen because patients now had to pay for the drug. The tests did not measure the patients' quality of life or look at whether they retained a measure of dignity. And like any statistical measure, particularly the result of the ADCS-ADL-severe test, the significance was so marginal that many patients very likely had no response at all. Statistical significance is crucial in science, but we also need to know exactly what measure achieved statistical significance and what is the impact of the drug's effect. And yet the result of a study like this one is that millions of individuals in nursing homes all over the country will now incur the added expense of taking donepezil at a cost of $150 a month. And families who decline the medication will incur the guilt of thinking that they have not done all that they could for their loved one.

The FDA standard for approving Alzheimer's disease drugs is that the drug sponsors must show evidence of two properties: (a) the drug must have a beneficial effect on one's cognitive function, such as through performance on memory tests or other neuropsychological puzzles; and (b) the drug must have a beneficial effect on how well one performs day-to-day activities. These effects are measured on standardized tests, and the scores on the tests are compared to control groups not on the drug or with individuals on the drug during an interval when not on the drug. Statisticians compare the scores using widely accepted methods, which determine whether any difference between the scores with and without the drug is significant. Significance means how likely is it that what might appear as a beneficial effect has actually occurred by chance. If the beneficial effect exceeds what one expects from chance, we say the effect is significant and the drug is on the road to approval, assuming no serious side effects occur. However, what remains missing is the magnitude of the beneficial effect. The actual benefit may be minimal, but whether the physician should use the drug falls outside the charge of the FDA and into the hands of the physician and, more important, the marketers in the companies that make the drug.

The FDA is not obligated, nor responsible by law, for determining the best medical practices physicians should pursue. The agency determines whether a drug is safe and effective by the guidelines laid out. The absence of regulation from the debate over best medical practice leaves the door open for drug companies to engage in marketing practices that create patient demand. Advertisements for an Alzheimer drug that depict a smiling grandpa next to his grown daughter convey many subtle and not so subtle messages that a good daughter will provide the drug regardless of its cost and regardless of how minimal its effects. In practice, how the drug will be used gets relegated to the insurers and other third-party payers who decide on whether the drug will be covered in their policies. This decision process is often opaque.

Not only do we pay high prices for drugs with modest effects, but we spend large sums on natural products that are also likely to have modest effects. All too often, research focuses on putting a patch on a problem rather than seeking real breakthroughs. Science is littered with examples of blind alleys and disappointing outcomes as by-products of the very nature of inquiry to push knowledge forward. But research dollars are sometimes directed at fads that are hot topics in the news but do not seem central to rooting out the cause of Alzheimer's.

After a popular groundswell developed around the use of the dietary supplement *Ginkgo biloba* to stave off cognitive decline, researchers decided to test it. In November 2008, the results of a $36.5 million, eight-year study of *Ginkgo biloba* were reported. The finding? *Ginkgo* is ineffective in reducing the development of dementia and Alzheimer's disease in older people. The research involved five branches of the National Institutes of Health—the National Center for Complementary and Alternative Medicine; the National Institute on Aging; the National Heart, Lung, and Blood Institute; the National Institute of Neurological Disorders and Stroke; and the Office of Dietary Supplements.

The study, known as GEM (Ginkgo Evaluation of Memory), enrolled 3,069 participants seventy-five years of age or older with normal cognition or mild cognitive impairment.[8] (Anyone with a diagnosis of dementia was excluded.) After screening, participants were randomly assigned to receive twice-daily doses of *Ginkgo* extract, or an identical sugar pill. The large study—which involved the University of Washington at Seattle, the University of Pittsburgh, Wake Forest University, Johns Hopkins University, and the University of California at Davis—followed the patients for an average of six years. During that time, 523 participants were diagnosed with dementia—246 in the placebo group and 277 in the *Ginkgo* group.

In other words, the use of *Gingko* had no overall effect. "We have made enormous progress in understanding the basic mechanisms involved in Alzheimer's disease, and we continue to pursue a vigorous program to translate what we know into the development and testing of new potential therapies for this devastating disease," Richard Hodes, MD, director of the National Institute of Aging, said at the time. "However, it is disappointing that the dietary supplement tested in this study had no effect in preventing Alzheimer's disease."[9]

For its part, the company that made the *Gingko* used in the study, Dr. Willmar Schwabe Pharmaceuticals in Karlsruhe, Germany, was not satisfied, saying it believes the GEM study results do not allow a final conclusion on the potential of the extract in dementia prevention.

The end result, after an investment of $36.5 million in research, remains the same: consumers should consult with their doctors and not rely on dietary supplements purchased over the counter.

BIOLOGICAL RESEARCH WILL CREATE A MEDICAL TREATMENT TIER AVAILABLE TO ONLY A SELECT FEW: HIGH MEDICAL COSTS ARE ABOUT TO SOAR

We begin with a very simple premise: Large pharmaceutical firms are mainly interested in drugs with benchmark profits of $1 billion or more. Development of a drug with a small market carries the same costs as one with a large market, and those costs must be recouped whether the number of potential customers is few or many. These companies assumed for a long time that to reach the billion-dollar mark, many people needed to purchase the medication to defray the costs. Only prevalent diseases that require lifelong treatment were attractive targets. So-called orphan diseases (those with relatively fewer sufferers) were ignored until the drug companies came along and demonstrated that it is possible to cash in if the price tag for these drugs is set high enough.

For example, for Avonex, used to treat multiple sclerosis, Biogen Idec Inc. charges $26,400 per year. However, to the credit of some companies, researchers have tackled several rare and fatal diseases. Genzyme Corporation has discovered an effective treatment for a form of Gaucher's disease (where fatty substances called lipids collect in the cells and organs) that affects fewer than 10,000 people worldwide. Gleevec (imatinib mesylate), approved by the FDA in 2001, targets a mutated protein in one type of leukemia, chronic myelogenous leukemia.

Taken to its logical conclusion, the economics of this thinking would hold that if even one person bought the drug and paid $1 billion per year, the drug development investment would be worth it and the company would have a "blockbuster." Suddenly, this option of treating smaller numbers of people at much higher prices came to make enormous sense to financial planners inside the big drug companies. After all, with few individuals being treated, rare side effects would diminish, the flawed one-size-fits-all philosophy could be abandoned in favor of high-end treatments tailored to the individual, and marketing costs would go down because a select group could be strategically targeted. In fact, through the Internet many self-organizing groups of families with rare diseases are springing up and becoming a collective voice for attention from the research community. As smaller genetically defined subgroups of patients are identified, there are smaller numbers of people for whom a medication might be appropriate. Those smaller numbers mean that costs must increase.

Treatment regimens with medication price tags in the $10,000 to $500,000 per year range are no longer unusual. Spending on specialty pharmaceuticals is now at $54 billion, or 20 percent of the entire pharmaceutical bill, and rising rapidly. Often, these top-shelf drugs fall into a category of medications called "biologics." These compounds generally have a larger molecular structure—think of the more complex molecular models you saw in chemistry class. They must be manufactured—a process chemists call being *synthesized*—by being grown inside an animal or in individual cells that are being kept alive in a laboratory.

The prime characteristic of these specialty drugs, however, is their stratospheric price tag. The claim that supposedly supports this high price is the high cost to discover and prepare these drugs. That claim is not dissimilar to the claim oil companies make that the high cost of searching and drilling for oil is what makes the price so high at the pump. What we do not hear from these companies is how much of the high price contributes to supporting record-high profit margins. How much of a company's profit is going back into new research beyond its allocated budget? How much of the research budget is directed toward discovery? It's not so easy to get the answers.

At this moment, all these issues are at the doorstep of anyone interested in Alzheimer's disease. Right now, most of the high-price drugs are used in cancer treatment, sometimes as the last option for an otherwise terminal patient. Among the first of these drugs is Avastin from Genentech Inc., a company in which the pharmaceutical giant Roche has a majority share, and Erbitux from ImClone Systems and another giant, Bristol-Myers Squibb. This specialty drug approach is now spreading to the Alzheimer field.

For example, significant resources have been put into the development of a biologic referred to as the Alzheimer's vaccine. In this approach, which originated with Dale Schenk, the chief scientific officer of Elan

Pharmaceuticals, headquartered in Dublin, Ireland, an antibody is infused and directed against the senile plaques. Just as an antibody directed against measles or mumps triggers the removal of the virus, the antibody against the amyloid protein should clean up the plaques. While this approach has encountered numerous setbacks, from serious side effects to questions of effectiveness, the investment goes on and the potential price tag, if the antibody drug comes to market, will be in the same range as other biologics. The lure for Pharma? Well, if one of the lead antibody drugs for Alzheimer's disease—Bapineuzumab—comes to market, it has the potential of $25 billion in annual sales worldwide, according to Linda Bannister, an Edward Jones analyst. If drugs for Alzheimer's disease come to the market, get ready for sticker shock.

The high cost of medications—in the $100,000 per year range per patient—will have an impact on the economics of physicians' practices and relationships with their patients. Usually, physicians write a prescription that gets filled at the pharmacy, but in the case of intravenous medications, the private physician must buy the drug up front. This method of payment means the physician holds the debt until paid back by the patient or the insurer. All too often, patients cannot afford their co-payment and insurers reject or delay their reimbursement. Writing in the *Wall Street Journal* on July 8, 2008, Marilyn Chase reported the story of Dr. Stephen Hufford, a San Francisco oncologist who incurred several hundred thousand dollars of debt while insurers delayed their payments. When he ordered $20,000 worth of chemotherapeutic drugs for three patients due in his office the next day, the distributor refused to deliver the medications unless he reduced his debt by $20,000 and paid for the order in advance. Dr. Hufford did not have $40,000 in his bank account. The thin string to which the treatment of these three patients was tied did not break in this case, because of Dr. Hufford's pleading with the company, but this situation will become more frequent. Favorable outcomes will become less and less frequent.

In this market, physicians are facing economic dilemmas for which they were never trained in medical school: they are having to reconcile cost with potential benefit. In cancer the benefit of these drugs is not a cure; it is extending life by as little as a few months. Likewise, an Alzheimer drug is also not likely to be a cure. In the case of cancer treatments, the financial exchange for those few months of extended life might be a child's college tuition. A survey reported in the *Journal of Clinical Oncology* by Deborah Schrag of the Dana-Farber Cancer Institute in Boston found that costs influenced treatment decisions among 23 percent of oncologists, and 16 percent of oncologists do not even discuss the high-priced options when they know the treatment would cause financial strain.[10] The clear implication is that if high-priced medications for Alzheimer's disease come to market, and they only slow disease progression, then doctors may not prescribe them. Physician liability in such cases has not yet been tested. In some European countries with state-run healthcare systems, governments have judged some treatments too expensive for the benefits they offer and have refused to pay for them.

THE OFF-LABEL QUAGMIRE AND THE COMPASSIONATE-USE QUICKSAND

Off-label drug use is what it sounds like: a doctor prescribes an FDA-approved drug for an unapproved condition. The practice is extremely common, and for some diseases, as much as half of all prescriptions are off-label. At first glance, off-label usage may not appear so perplexing. The practice is perfectly legal for physicians, but laden with legal and ethical issues for drug companies. No one disputes this distinction as a reasonable starting point. Certainly, no one wants a drug marketed for use against a disease before it has been rigorously tested. But neither do people want to tie the hands of the physician who may find a drug useful under special circumstances.

One of the most notorious examples of off-label use involved the drug Gabapentin, which was approved by the FDA for adjunctive therapy in treatment of partial seizures and neuralgia. Among the off-label uses reported were bipolar disorder, peripheral neuropathy, diabetic neuropathy, complex regional pain syndrome, attention deficit disorder, restless leg syndrome, trigeminal neuralgia, periodic limb movement disorder of sleep, migraine headaches, and alcohol withdrawal syndrome. As sales of Gabapentin for off-label uses soared, legal concerns arose. While off-label prescriptions are common for some drugs and are perfectly legal (if not always appropriate), marketing of off-label uses of a drug is strictly illegal. Furthermore, "off-label" prescriptions for Gabapentin were often not the optimal treatment.[11] On May 13, 2004, Pfizer pleaded guilty to criminal violation of the Federal Food, Drug, and Cosmetic Act and paid a criminal fine of $240 million for its involvement in marketing the drug. Although the legal distinctions between physician and drug company regarding off-label use may seem clear, when the physician prescribes a drug for an off-label use, a lingering suspicion may remain that a pharmaceutical company is pushing its product.

Attempting to get an off-label use for a drug paid for by an insurance company is an obstacle course. These are gray zones where the interests of different parties seem to color the apparently straightforward matter of getting the most effective medication possible for the condition.

For Alzheimer's disease, off-label use is very relevant. No one knows when a drug intended for one use could prove beneficial for Alzheimer's patients. Dozens of medications slated for other uses have been studied for use in Alzheimer's disease, and peer-reviewed articles in reputable journals report these findings, some of them favorable. Drugs in many categories are on this list, including statins, normally used for heart patients, antihypertensives intended for remedying blood pressure problems, antiepileptics intended to control seizures, and anti-inflammatory drugs designed to control various types of swelling in the body, as well as more obscure off-label remedies such as IVIg (intravenous immune globulin, designed for immune system deficiencies) and methylene blue, an old drug intended for urinary tract infections. Informed patients may request these medications, and physicians who have studied the evidence may be tempted to offer them.

But what constitutes sufficient information to prescribe a drug off-label for an unintended condition like Alzheimer's? And where does that information come from? Directly from the drug company? Certainly not. It often comes from a drug representative who is distributing information that has actually been published by someone from outside the drug company. Here, then, is one of the many gray zones. Discussing the busy internist without time to read medical articles or package inserts, Peter Pitts, president of the Center for Medicines in the Public Interest (CMPI, New York) was quoted as saying, "They [physicians] are learning information anecdotally through patients and colleagues at conferences and through conversations with Pharma reps. And when it comes to having reps hand a physician a reprint of a medical article that discusses an off-label use, I think it clearly and unambiguously falls under the safe harbor of the free and fair dissemination of information."[12] To protect against biased information, Jerry Avorn at the Harvard Medical School has championed counterdetailing, which uses the methods of drug reps—direct visits to doctor's offices—to present balanced knowledge by independent experts.[13]

Off-label use of medications in the area of impaired ability to reason, understand, and remember is precisely an arena in which the approaches to information described in chapter 8 are applicable. Patients with Alzheimer's disease and their families frequently request off-label medications and often come armed with supporting evidence that they have downloaded from the Internet, or gleaned from friends, or read about in the press. We need to pool the experience of many individuals who are using medications for undesignated purposes through central, independent Web sites to which physicians will have ready access when making the tough decisions about whether to agree to patient requests for an off-label medication.

A few years ago, the husband of one of my patients with Alzheimer's disease learned from a Web search that a purified mixture of human antibodies administered intravenously called IVIg might be effective in Alzheimer's disease. He requested IVIg and had the means to pay for its high cost as well as for a nurse to come to his home and administer it. IVIg has been proven safe and effective in several immune system disorders, but was not approved in Alzheimer's disease, although studies are under way to verify the initial report of effectiveness discovered on the Web by my patient's husband. I had been aware of the early report and believed that Norman Relkin, the physician from Weill Cornell Medical College in New York City, who first reported on IVIg for Alzheimer's disease, is a reliable and distinguished investigator. However, brief reports that claim effectiveness for various off-label drugs are frequent, and I do not generally offer these drugs to patients. However, in this case the patient's husband, who cared for her with extraordinary devotion, who tracked down every possible lead, and who walked with her every morning to review the names of the trees on their property, intended to leave no stone unturned in his quest to get the medication. A colleague of mine, Dr. Brad Joseph, and I offered her the medication.

Looking back on the treatment, the patient's disease did not progress for the nearly two years on the medication, but the significance of a single anecdotal experience is nil because some Alzheimer patients stabilize for a few years without any treatment. In this sense, we did not add to medical knowledge and without demonstrated effectiveness we might not have accomplished anything whatsoever. We provided an experimental treatment that would be prohibitively expensive to most other people. Did the family wealth give them privileged access to slowing the ravages of Alzheimer's disease or did their wealth make them susceptible to being a human guinea pig? How are we to be guided in the use of off-label medications? Perhaps the ancient physician guideline—*primum non nocere*, first do no harm—is the best guideline. Justification for off-label use—most common in cancer—is that the patient is terminal without any other options. Alzheimer is also a terminal disease without meaningful treatment options. Certainly, a case can be made for the compassionate use of medications in Alzheimer's disease as long as there is ethical oversight.

EMPLOYER COVERAGE WILL REQUIRE LIFESTYLE CHANGES TO REDUCE RISK

Imagine showing up at your neurologist's office one afternoon with a diagnosis of early Alzheimer's disease and being told that your insurance will not cover your visit because you did not live right. Before you even get to see the doctor, the person at the desk regretfully informs you that your dietary excess, TV on the couch instead of on the treadmill, and the invitations you shunned that would have enriched your social life have all come due. Your coverage has been terminated because you did not take personal responsibility to stave off disease. Increasingly, we are seeing that people are held responsible for the consequences of their bad health habits.

It begins quite benignly. One day at the office you are offered free admission to the health club next door. The next day the cafeteria offerings are more limited on the dessert counter. As the payer for your health insurance, the company wants to keep you healthy and is encouraging you to do so. For now. Next, encouragement becomes mandatory compliance.

The cost of medical insurance will factor in the added risk of lifestyle decisions known to contribute to certain diseases. Risks such as smoking are often already factored in. This eat-broccoli-drop-your-premium approach to health insurance is the remedy of choice in some places where healthcare costs are soaring. As the data accrue that lifestyle can greatly affect one's chances of getting Alzheimer's disease, will third-party payers extract consequences from those who indulge themselves?

Lisa Takeuchi Cullen, a writer for *Time* magazine, is one of many bringing national attention to this new twist on the problem of personal freedom and who pays for healthcare. In an article on March 24, 2008, she noted that employer responsibility for health insurance dates from the time of Franklin D. Roosevelt, who did not include healthcare in his New Deal. Instead, employers were encouraged to offer private health insurance to workers through tax breaks, labor restrictions, and accounting rules. Privatized health insurance looked like another jewel in the crown for the American system until healthcare costs began to hit the stratosphere. In 2005, healthcare expenditures were pegged at $2 trillion. The contribution from employers to employee healthcare expenditures shrank from 48 percent in 1960 to 15 percent in 2000. Many unpalatable solutions came along, including managed care, high-deductible plans, and health savings accounts.

Physicians feel stifled and boxed-in by large bureaucracies. Private insurance companies, on the one hand, and the government-run Medicare system on the other, determine how much a doctor will be paid to treat a patient. Doctors receive the highest fees for procedures, such as surgery or MRI scans—but an Alzheimer's patient, once diagnosed, could live for years without needing such treatment. Simpler, more direct methods of communicating with patients, such as e-mail, are not reimbursed. Drugs that came on the market with high expectations have not proven to be highly effective for Alzheimer's patients—and the drug development process is long, complex, and expensive, even for the largest pharmaceutical companies.

Most of our potential impact on Alzheimer's disease lies in the area of prevention—and allowing doctors the time and space (and fee structure) to practice preventive medicine should be a key point of any healthcare reform program.

NOTES

1. A. Catlin et al., the National Health Expenditure Accounts Team, "National Health Spending in 2005: The Slowdown Continues," *Health Affairs* 26 (2007): 142–53. In addition, see M. R. Nuwer et al., "The US Health Care System," *Neurology* 71 (2008): 1907–13. For more on private insurance and overhead costs, see "Proposal of the Physicians' Working Group for Single-Payer National Health Insurance," *Journal of the American Medical Association* 290 (2003): 798–805.

2. S. Maxwell, S. Zuckerman, and R. A. Berenson, "Procedure-Driven Care," *New England Journal of Medicine* 356, no. 18 (May 3, 2007): 1853–61.

3. White paper available at http://www.ama-assn.org/ama/upload/mm/363/pliwhitepaper.pdf.

4. Joseph Antos, "Have Health Reformers Forgotten Medicare?" *Health Policy Outlook*, American Enterprise Institute online, July 8, 2008; "The Sustainable Growth Rate Formula for Setting Medicare's Physician Payment Rates," *CBO Economic and Budget Issue Brief*, September 6, 2006.

5. B. Winblad et al., "Donepezil in Patients with Severe Alzheimer's Disease: Double-Blind, Parallel-Group, Placebo-Controlled Study," *Lancet* 367, no. 9516 (2006): 1057–65.

6. Stephanie Cajigal, "FDA Approves Donepezil For Severe Dementia—

Experts Question Why," *Neurology Today* 6, no. 22 (November 21, 2006): 1–8.

7. Ibid

8. S. T. DeKosky et al., "Ginkgo Biloba for Prevention of Dementia," Ginkgo Evaluation of Memory Study, *Journal of the American Medical Association* 300, no. 19 (2008): 2253–62.

9. Ibid

10. D. Schrag and M. Hanger, "Medical Oncologists' Views on Communicating with Patients about Chemotherapy Costs: A Pilot Survey," *Journal of Clinical Oncology* 25, no. 2 (January 10, 2007): 233–37.

11. A. Mack, "Evidence-Based Use of Gabapentin," *Journal of Managed Care Pharmacy* 9, no. 6 (2003): 559–68.

12. Pitts quote from http://www.cmpi.org/.

13. Mark Ratner and Trisha Gura, "Off-Label or Off-Limits?" *Nature Biotechnology* 26 (2008): 867.

7

COGNITIVE IMPAIRMENT AND DECISION MAKING

I WAKE and feel the fell of dark, not day.
What hours, O what black hours we have spent
This night! what sights you, heart, saw; ways you went!
And more must, in yet longer light's delay.
    With witness I speak this. But where I say
Hours I mean years, mean life. And my lament
Is cries countless, cries like dead letters sent
To dearest him that lives alas! away.
    —GERARD MANLEY HOPKINS, *POEMS OF GERARD MANLEY HOPKINS*

WHY DO PEOPLE WHO ARE STRONGLY OPPOSED TO RECEIVING TOTAL CARE OFTEN END UP RECEIVING TOTAL CARE IF THEY BECOME DEMENTED?

Many people say they would rather not go on living than accept total care because of severe cognitive impairment. They might say they prefer to conclude their life with dignity and without becoming a burden on others. Despite these wishes, the great majority of those who become demented seem to lose control over their fate and either accept a total-care setting or slip into it involuntarily. The reasons that underlie this paradox are not understood.

Perhaps those who say they would prefer to die, rather than live with moderate to severe dementia, change their mind about dying as

179

they become impaired. Or they may remain firm in their commitment, but choosing the moment of action has become an insurmountable obstacle. Or perhaps they retain the resolve to end their life, but when the time comes, they no longer have the mental capacity to implement their wishes. Taking one's life involves some planning. That very sort of planning—involving strategy to set out step-by-step future action—is an area of cognition called "executive function," a capacity that is frequently damaged in Alzheimer's disease. Some people may not act on the desire to avoid total care because family members prefer to see them alive, even though they are a mere shadow of their former selves, rather than not see them at all. And many people may feel a deep moral conviction based on their religion that prevents them from hastening a natural death. All these possibilities rely on patients who have enough cognitive capacity to reach a decision about their own lives.

The mother of a friend of mine, in her eighties, opted to take her own life when she learned that she began to have the earliest symptoms of Alzheimer's disease. She set for herself a limit on the amount of forgetting she would tolerate, and when she reached that level she put on a recording of an opera that she adored, placed a rose by her bed, dressed up, and took a lethal overdose of a medication that she had saved for this occasion. She had previously discussed her decision with her children (her husband was deceased), and when the time came she called them to be with her at the conclusion of her life. They came, and to this day, as they are approaching her age, they continue to have enormous admiration for the brave and dignified decision she made. None of them viewed her decision as selfish or nihilistic. But these views are not universally shared, and we must have room in our stance on these issues for those who strongly disagree with taking one's life. After all, we might legitimately ask whether the woman in the story was mistaken and did not have Alzheimer's disease or maybe her doctor was wrong about the diagnosis, or suppose, most nefariously, her children wished her death for financial gain and coerced their mother's decision either directly or by innuendo. The entire topic is so sensitive that it has been kept under wraps and any attempt to begin a conversation at the national level gets drowned in the powerful emotions that surround the issues.

For those who have thought out the complexities and favor a framework for thinking about the problem, the now defunct Hemlock Society (which after several iterations changed its name to Compassion and Choices) offered a philosophy based on the death of Socrates. In its literature, Compassion and Choices points out that Socrates' death, in 329 BCE, after being sentenced to death or a lonely barren exile, occurred only after he had discussed these options for hours with his friends. His decision to drink the hemlock was self-chosen and arrived at rationally. For us the analogy to exile on a barren island is terminal illness, and Socrates made a personal choice to hasten his death rather than live in misery.

But Socrates did not face the problem of timing his death—the timetable was set by the court. Timing one's death within a window of competence is difficult, and the ability to do the deed can easily slip by. It is not an easy decision, of course. Various "right-to-die" organizations have voiced powerful arguments in favor of helping people of sound mind who have deeply considered the issues and opt to end their lives.

Experiencing a change of heart about taking one's own life certainly does not require the added complication of dementia. The story of Thomas Wilson, the central character in "The Lotus Eater" by William Somerset Maugham, is an example.[1] At age thirty-five, he quit his job as a banker and used all of his savings to purchase a twenty-five-year annuity that provided him with sufficient funds to live comfortably on the island of Capri. He had reasoned that the deal he struck with himself—twenty-five years of happiness—was a fair exchange for ending his life at sixty. Maugham then points out that there was a flaw in Wilson's plan:

> It had never occurred to him that after twenty-five years of complete happiness, in this quiet backwater, with nothing in the world to disturb his serenity, his character would gradually lose its strength. The will needs obstacles in order to exercise its power; when it is never thwarted, when no effort is needed to achieve one's desires, because one has placed one's desires only in the things that can be obtained by stretching out one's hand, the will grows impotent. If you walk on a level all the time the muscles you need to climb a mountain will atrophy. These observations are trite, but there they are. When Wilson's annuity expired he had no longer the resolution to make the end, which was the price he had agreed to pay for that long period of happy tranquility. I do not think, as far as I could gather, both from what my friend told me and afterwards from others, that he wanted courage. It was just that he couldn't make up his mind. He put it off from day to day.

A real-life case of facing these issues is that of Thomas Grayboys, a renowned Boston cardiologist who described his ordeal with a dementing illness similar to Alzheimer's disease called Lewy body dementia.[2] Even as his disease advanced and his memory lapses and disorientation became obvious, he continued to practice medicine while friends and staff were reluctant to confront him directly. Not until

2005, about seven years into the disease, did his partners tell him to retire. Although Grayboys explicitly states in his book *Life in the Balance* that he does not want to be kept alive "with a mind erased," he also states, "no matter how much we intellectualize and plan for the day when a critical life-and-death decision will have to be made, when that day comes all bets are off."

A cognitively intact person is quite appropriately allowed full control over his or her fate. However, these difficult issues become even more complex in the face of dementia, when the ability to communicate gradually declines over several years. Patients with cancer, whose mental faculties are often intact until they die, sometimes reach a point when they concede that the ravages and pain of the disease, combined with the fading hope of recovery, make it reasonable to hasten the end. A discussion about end-of-life options remains possible. The person makes clear his wishes to the family and may have even prepared documents that detail the circumstances under which he would desire life support or prefer withholding life support. The hospice movement was born from this thinking. In the case of severe brain injury, an active person may suddenly become comatose and can no longer discuss end-of-life options. But the abrupt transition leaves as our only reference point a vibrant individual who may have been quite clear about her wishes for or against life support. In some cases, there may be an advance directive that informs the doctor about the kind of care desired if one becomes unable to make medical decisions, such as after falling into a coma. A good advance directive defines acceptable treatments under a variety of scenarios related to how sick one is and the chances of recovery.

The situation is full of ambiguities in Alzheimer's disease. Decisions are inordinately more complicated because the person is right there in front of you.

The planning for death involves a living person, a person who seems to be there, but not quite; a person with whom it is hard to come away and feel like every word of the conversation was understood even though a conversation did take place. How much meaning can one attribute to a nod of the head or to a simple utterance, a yes or a no, in the absence of any discussion, is never clear. The person is like a puzzle with missing pieces. Family members or caregivers feel compelled to draw conclusions from nothing more than a gesture or a sense of recognition in the person's eyes. We may be flummoxed by normal social mores, which do not meet any legal standard. Under normal circumstances, uncertainties are filled in by assumptions, and if there is goodwill, these assumptions are usually correct. In the case of Alzheimer's disease, we are required to fill in more and more, and the chances that our assumptions are correct about what the affected person may desire decline accordingly.

Alzheimer's disease takes its toll over the years. During this prolonged period, patients who clearly state that they never want to live in the terminal stages of Alzheimer's disease and would prefer to die lose the ability to execute or convey their wishes. There are advance directives and healthcare power of attorney forms that can be completed, but some healthy elders put off filling them out. Once cognitive decline sets in, the transition to impaired communication is slow and fragmented in the sense that along the way many partial states exist in which the affected individual may do slightly better or worse from moment to moment. The time for action inexorably slips away. A harsh existential duality comes into play. When a patient can take action, he may not want to. At the time when he wants to take action, he may not be able to.

APATHY REPLACES DESPONDENCY

Well before communication is lost, a person with dementia may lose resolve about ending life due to apathy. Apathy has replaced despondency. The individual gives only fleeting consideration to her compromised state, but most of the time she is no longer dwelling on herself. One of the saddest comments ever made to me by an Alzheimer patient was her complaint about what was most uncomfortable for her. With an overwhelming sense of resignation, she said, "I have nothing to think about." Thought is an involuntary activity that travels about without regard for either time or place. While riding on the bus we might travel back to the schoolyard of our childhood. Or we can land for the umpteenth time in the same dispute we just had with our spouse, revisiting the same words over and over. Or we can project forward to what summering in Tuscany might be like.

Thought travels at odd angles through nearly instantaneous transitions. Thought is the inner workings of our mind, which fabricate our identities. The time spent in thought serves to build and sustain the content that we package together as an identity. As the time devoted to thought drains away, so does our identity. In this view, the entire dilemma over continuing to live disappears from one's subjective, perceptual universe. To feel concern about a loss, we require the memory of its former presence. Without a memory trace, what we've lost becomes no different than what we never had. No one feels any loss about not being able to see behind his head because whatever scene lies there has never been a part of our visual field. But lose a piece of the visual field that lies to the right or to the left in front of us and we are continuously reminded of its absence.

Concern about one's fate is a particularly human trait, which might vanish when we have no memory of the recent past when we were pre-occupied with our fate. We've lost, but may not miss, may not even be aware of, this former preoccupation. Of course, the vanishing of iden-tity does wipe out emotion. A person may feel wonderful in the moment to see a familiar face, but not be able to long for the person when he or she is not there. A person in this state can experience fear, which is more immediate, but may be less prone to abstract worries that bring about anxiety.

A more detailed brain effort is required to stitch together an imag-ined future. The ability to perform such mental projections and con-ceptualize death may be greatly blunted. The near impossibility of having a conversation with a loved one about advance directives or has-tening death is the end-of-life issue peculiar to the Alzheimer setting.

How troubling to be faced with the prospect of needing total care, of not even being aware of the indignities through which one is suf-fering. Because a person in this state is no longer capable of conveying his wishes, we quite appropriately err on the side of providing all the care needed to maintain the comfort of the individual. But the conver-sation we refuse to have is a discussion of our options—before we lose our self-generated aura of what we consider as our identity. While our predictive acumen is improving rapidly—more and more we know far in advance who is likely to get Alzheimer's disease—any discussion about ending our lives somewhere in the course of the decline remains covert, uncomfortable, and shrouded in stigma.

PREDICTING ALZHEIMER'S DISEASE

The discussion must begin with how we know who will get the disease, how accurate our prediction is, and how we can predict when the disease will occur. In rare cases of Alzheimer's disease like those described in chapter 1, we can predict with near certainty whether a member of the family will get the disease. The test is a simple genetic analysis of blood or saliva. Predicting when the person will get the disease if she has one of these severe mutations is not as accurate, but the age of onset is often similar within a family. However, the age at which the person may show symptoms of the disease may differ among different families who carry closely related genetic mutations. Families that harbor these mutations are increasingly taking a strong stand on the measures they will and will not accept to prolong life—see the chapter 1 comments by Julie Lawson.

Among the vast majority of people destined to get sporadic Alzheimer's disease—not those with rare genetic mutations—predictive testing is more challenging. No test rivals the genetic predictions of the dominant Alzheimer mutations, which carry their blindingly clear message of doom in the DNA from the time of conception. Nevertheless, the ability to anticipate sporadic Alzheimer's disease many years before dementia occurs is improving rapidly. One common risk factor is another genetic marker called APOE. This gene was also discussed in chapter 1. Suffice it to say here that a positive APOE test is not like the other early onset familial Alzheimer genes. While carriers of the APOE4 mutation definitely have an increased risk, getting the disease is not a foregone conclusion as it is with the other gene mutations. A positive APOE test has to be weighed with many other factors in its interpretation. In addition to APOE mutations, the greatest genetic risk for late onset of the disease, other genes appear to play a minor role in disease risk.

All genetic testing falls into a unique category because the test results do not change over a lifetime. The risk that a mutant gene carries for getting a disease may change, depending on other environmental factors or other genes that may improve or aggravate the effects of the mutation. But the mutation in the DNA is irrevocable. It is there for life. It's crucially important to be crystal clear that having a mutation by no means implies that one has the disease. Even a carrier of one of the powerful early onset Alzheimer disease mutations does not have the disease until his brain starts to show signs of degeneration and he starts to become clinically demented. Before this time, he is only a mutation carrier and not affected by the disease. All other types of testing that do not involve genes only test for the earliest signs of the disease.

Tests that look for early signs of the disease fall into two categories—those that rely on paper-and-pencil neuropsychological testing of the patient and those that attempt to visualize early Alzheimer changes in the brain. Paper-and-pencil testing has given rise to the concept of mild cognitive impairment, or MCI. In contrast to Alzheimer's, MCI does not mean a person will not be able to carry out the important activities that comprise daily life. It is merely a test score, corrected for age and measured against others who have taken the test. Other than what can be discerned by formal testing, no problems with memory or with carrying out the tasks of daily living may be apparent. Highly specific criteria for the diagnosis of MCI have not been established, and how well it predicts the eventual development of Alzheimer's disease is still not clear. However, MCI, particularly memory loss, does confer a significantly increased risk of developing Alzheimer's disease and may be considered an early symptom of the disease.

Brain imaging also carries inherent ambiguities. As described in chapter 2, it is now possible to visualize the amyloid in the senile plaques of a living individual. This discovery represents an important step for the field, but early indicators from this testing have questioned the association between the existence of amyloids and the disease. While the significance of directly seeing Alzheimer brain features needs further clarification, it is likely that the presence of amyloid found by brain imaging will indicate an increased risk of getting the disease. In fact, even before these brain-imaging techniques were available it was known that the amyloid deposits begin at least a decade and maybe two decades before any symptoms were detectable. So while we do not know whether all people with senile plaques but no apparent symptoms will eventually contract Alzheimer's disease, the presence of these plaques may be enough to prompt more aggressive intervention, such as removing the plaques with an antibody-type drug described as described in chapter 3.

Taken together, Alzheimer's testing is closing in on early signs and refining our accuracy in diagnosis. Assuming we can have in advance a fairly good idea whether we will get the disease, might we want to put more effort into detailing our wishes for an end-of-life scenario that includes Alzheimer's disease? Although predictive testing is increasingly improving early diagnosis, now the average time from diagnosis to death in patients with Alzheimer's disease is ten years. During this interval, interest in the patient's ongoing welfare by the medical establishment wanes rapidly. So a ten-year period opens during which time patients and their families are searching for information about treatment, desperately inquiring about promising experimental leads, patching together a support system, and generally not fully facing the future.

The irrefutable fact is that all patients who receive the diagnosis of Alzheimer's disease face the inevitable need for assistance with every aspect of daily living. But who is talking about the available options for those who do not want total care, those who would prefer to end their lives rather than receive total care? The subject is so uncomfortable that public and private discussion has been muted. The inherent optimism of human beings, the uncomfortable nature of the topic, and societal norms all conspire to prevent this discussion. As long as the topic is swept under the rug, the total-care industry can thrive and people will clamor for more subsidies to pay industry providers to create environments where those with severe Alzheimer's disease can subsist. The demand for total care represents an opportunity to the providers of these services as long as we sustain the perception of the need. Nevertheless, the time for this discussion is now because predictive testing for Alzheimer's disease is becoming increasingly accurate and increasingly available.

In the near term, many individuals will know they face the prospect of an incurable brain disease that will leave them in need of help with nearly every activity of daily living. As the number of people who know their fate grows, what voices will we hear among them? What viewpoints, what philosophies, what actions? What social changes lie on the horizon? Clearly, cultural factors will play a role in everyone's thinking about these issues, so assessments need to take into account the cultural setting of the subject. As people become more comfortable with the topic, elders may be able to face their future in a manner that is both realistic and at least partially free from the grip of fear.

PHYSICIAN-ASSISTED SUICIDE RULES ARE NOT APPLICABLE TO ALZHEIMER'S DISEASE

Perhaps the best starting point for this vexing issue is the medical-ethical territory that is opened by the problem of physician-assisted suicide. This term refers to a practice in which the physician, at the request of the patient, provides a lethal dose of medication, which the patient intends to use to end his or her own life. Perhaps most important, physician-assisted suicide is not euthanasia because the patient, not the physician, administers the lethal medication. Physician-assisted suicide is illegal in all states except Oregon. Another end-of-life practice is terminal sedation, in which a terminally ill patient is sedated to the point of unconsciousness and then allowed to die of the disease, starvation, or dehydration. Terminal sedation borders on providing a patient with a dosage of medication that impairs respiration and thus may hasten death. In most cases, this practice has been upheld in court decisions and supported by professional medical societies. Even broader support exists for allowing a competent patient to refuse or withdraw life-sustaining treatment.

One can immediately recognize that everything from the terminology used to the practices themselves will need to be rethought when applied to Alzheimer's disease. The biggest conflict for the ethical boundaries of physician-assisted suicide is that once the person is beyond a certain point in the Alzheimer disease process, he is no longer competent and may not be able to self-administer a lethal dose of medication. Another area of conflict is that some definitions of a terminal condition require that the death be likely in six months, which is not the case for Alzheimer's disease. However, the ethical debate around physician-assisted suicide does resonate with some of the Alzheimer-related issues. For example, some ethicists argue that physician-assisted suicide is a rational choice for a person who seeks to escape unbearable suffering. How much Alzheimer patients suffer is not clear. Some may be in pain but unable to communicate their pain. Whether an environment of total care and its reflection on one's dignity is suffering is debatable. Nevertheless, the argument in favor of physician-assisted suicide relies on individual liberty and the right of a competent person to choose for himself the course of his life, including its end. Certainly, that is a right we do not want to deny to Alzheimer patients. As a consequence of treating physician-assisted suicide as illegal, we have also stifled such critical discussion.

The discussion needs to include both sides of the issue. The most vocal among those opposed to physician-assisted suicide put forth a sanctity-of-life argument. However, proponents of physician-assisted suicide also believe in the sanctity of life, and under circumstances that are no longer tenable as a way to live, the sanctity of life may serve as the kernel of their argument to hasten its end. The growing interest in the concept of a "good death" might be viewed as part of the sanctity of life. Although we have a lot to learn about what is a good death and how individuals may differ in their view of a good death, almost certainly a medical death is not a good death. Pneumonia, which at one time was called an "old man's friend" because it was a peaceful way to die, is now often aggressively treated with powerful antibiotics.

A more serious opposing argument is the potential for abuse. Geronticide, or the euthanasia of elders simply because they are old and are perceived to have outlived their utility to society, is not only cruel and selfish but also criminal and flagrantly immoral. Although folk literature is full of kindhearted customs, such as removing roof tiles or opening windows to provide the departing soul an easier exit, or taking away a dying person's pillow, or cutting a scrap from one's clothing—all of these were usually intended as a salve to ease the transition toward death. Unfortunately, history more commonly reveals a harsher scenario for terminating the old and feeble.

Historic abuse is particularly powerful in the context of Alzheimer's disease, with the specter that physician-assisted suicide will serve as a cost-cutting measure to rein in the astronomical costs of care for the demented. Or physician-assisted suicide might be excessively used among people who cannot afford more expensive care settings. Financially burdened family members might put undue pressure on a terminally ill person to request physician-assisted suicide. Furthermore, if a mistake is made—for example, perhaps the condition may turn out not to be terminal—suicide cannot be reversed. Nevertheless, surveys of practicing physicians show that about 20 percent of them receive a request for physician-assisted suicide sometime in their career, and this number is most likely an underestimate.

The poignancy and immediacy of these issues is evident in the health reform debate today. On one side we hear the concern of facing years of prolonged indignity, of a life without one's mind, and feeling like a burden to one's family. On the other side we hear the danger of slipping closer to coercion in hastening the end of elders. Some individuals will say I want the freedom to decide how my life will end, and if that ending requires some form of suicide, I do not want the hand of government to limit my options. Others will say I want the assurance that I can live all the years I was given, and even in a feeble state life is not an indignity, and the government must not create the means by which social pressures arise that lead me to accept curtailing my life despite my reluctance. Instead of taking this serious debate to hysterical levels with notions like "death panels," which we now hear in the health reform chatter, we need to raise the level of the conversation. We need to search for the assurances that will definitively prevent coercion of elders to opt for death and be sure that in questionable cases we always err on the side of life. At the same time, we need to find a path for those who do not want to spend their final days in the grip of a total-care facility and give them the freedom to end life with dignity while still in possession of their intellect.

END-OF-LIFE ISSUES FOR ALZHEIMER'S DISEASE PATIENTS: THE NEED FOR A NEW ETHICAL LANDSCAPE

Individuals with Alzheimer's disease, particularly those with moderate and advanced disease, fall far outside the boundaries that surround current thinking about the rules of physician-assisted suicide. New thinking is needed to address end-of-life issues associated with Alzheimer's disease. However, the problem itself is by no means new. The irony of dementia as the conclusion of life has been treated for centuries as part of the human condition. William Shakespeare described seven stages of life in *As You Like It*:

> All the world's a stage,
> And all the men and women merely players:
> They have their exits and their entrances;
> And one man in his time plays many parts,
> His acts being seven ages. At first the infant,
> Mewling and puking in the nurse's arms.
> Then the whining school-boy, with his satchel
> And shining morning face, creeping like snail
> Unwillingly to school. And then the lover,
> Sighing like furnace, with a woeful ballad
> Made to his mistress' eyebrow. Then a soldier,
> Full of strange oaths, and bearded like the pard,
> Jealous in honor, sudden and quick in quarrel,
> Seeking the bubble reputation
> Even in the cannon's mouth. And then the justice,
> In fair round belly with good capon lined,
> With eyes severe and beard of formal cut,
> Full of wise saws and modern instances;
> And so he plays his part. The sixth age shifts
> Into the lean and slipper'd pantaloon,
> With spectacles on nose and pouch on side,
> His youthful hose, well saved, a world too wide
> For his shrunk shank; and his big manly voice,
> Turning again toward childish treble, pipes
> And whistles in his sound. Last scene of all,
> That ends this strange eventful history,
> Is second childishness and mere oblivion,
> Sans teeth, sans eyes, sans taste, sans everything.[3]

Jacob and Wilhelm Grimm in their tale called the "The Duration of Life" told how in the interest of equality God gave all creatures equal lifespans of thirty years.[4] But the animals pleaded with God to shorten their allotted time. The ass spoke about years of carrying a heavy load, the dog complained that in his final years he could only run from corner to corner unable to bark and without teeth for biting, and the monkey said, "I am always supposed to be playing funny tricks and making faces so people will laugh, but when they give me an apple and I bite into it, it is always sour. How often is sorrow hidden behind a joke." So

God reduced all their lifespans. Man, on the other hand, thought thirty years too brief. So God gave him all the unwanted years of the ass, the dog, and the monkey, which brought his lifespan to seventy. For his first thirty years man is happy. Then come the years from the ass when one burden after another is laid upon him. Afterward comes the dog's final years when he lies in the corner growling, without teeth, unable to bite. Finally, he spends the monkey's final years weak-headed and foolish and doing silly things that become a laughingstock for children.

To begin to tackle this complex problem, we must break it down because the approach will differ depending on the circumstances. Consider the cognitively normal individual who knows she will develop the disease and does not want to spend her final years in total care. Or consider the person who already has Alzheimer's dementia and family members have reason to believe that the affected individual would not want total care. The two cases entail vastly different issues. Or break it down another way. A person is faced with the need for total care to survive—are there options short of suicide to avoid this fate or shorten the time spent in total care? The common starting point for all these considerations is a sincere and open discussion that always puts the wishes of the individual first. Some sense of who among family and friends belongs at the table should be a topic from the beginning. Whether the issue at hand is predictive testing or prognosis of existing disease, the accuracy and the limitations of medical knowledge must be absolutely clear.

The discussion around options once a person requires help with activities of daily living is essentially how much assistance will the person accept and what medical interventions are acceptable when a medical problem arises. For most people, palliative care to alleviate pain only is acceptable once a person has minimal mobility, can no longer communicate, and can no longer feed him- or herself. However, each condition requires a decision. The most common conditions that occur are infections. After a discussion about the wishes of the patient and the medical condition, one might decide not to treat pneumonia, but a urinary tract infection that might cause painful urination could be treated. Another frequent medical intervention is the use of a blood thinner to diminish the likelihood of clot formation in the legs or heart should its rhythm become irregular. Blood thinners are not without their own complications, particularly hemorrhaging if the patient is bruised or cut. Whether to withhold a blood thinner is another decision. Some interventions require transfer of the individual from an assisted living facility to a hospital, and the family may decline the transfer. The overriding guideline is the comfort of the individual, which is the whole point of palliative care. If the patient is uncomfortable because he is short of breath, the preferred option might be sedation, rather than an extensive diagnostic workup to address the lung malfunction.

The situation becomes more difficult when the request is made to withhold feeding from a person who can no longer feed himself. Hastening death in this manner still falls in the realm of withholding life-sustaining support, but it is no longer a medical matter that has arisen around a precipitous situation, such as an inability to breathe without assistance. The key staff from whom one needs support are no longer the physicians, but the nursing staff and the many foot soldiers who tend to the severely debilitated. For many people, no longer feeding the person, and withholding a feeding tube, is the kindest measure that can be taken to end an otherwise hopeless condition. The patient may have expressed this wish many times and the family may concur. But the nursing staff may not agree. And so the big question about whether we can ask health professionals to carry out legal requests to which they are morally opposed comes into play.

Julie Lawson, whose family has been ravaged by early onset Alzheimer's disease, says that end-of-life questions are crucial. After her experience with her sister—the family decided on no feeding tube, and wanted her to be able to die in relative peace surrounded by loved ones—she built end-of-life discussions into her search for a nursing home for her brother, Butch, who has also been diagnosed with the disease. Because Julie and Butch discussed so many aspects of the care for their sisters Fran and Maureen, Julie knows that Butch would not want to extend his life if he cannot feed himself, or swallow. She knows full well that she will need help, and she will make arrangements with visiting nurses and hospice when the time comes.

If we can reach an accord on withholding food, and perhaps water under some circumstances, the next consideration is whether one can take a more active role in hastening the death of someone who is in a vegetative state because of Alzheimer's disease. This brand of dilemma is of great interest to ethicists, philosophers, and most recently to neuroethicists, who can observe the brain activity of those making momentous decisions on a functional MRI scanner. The analogous decision-making process is the famous trolley car problem: A trolley is running out of control down a track with five people tied to the track directly ahead. The driver has just had a heart attack, but you can flip a switch that will send the trolley down a different track, where a single person is tied to that track. Do you flip the switch? The question hinges on the importance we place on taking an active role in causing a death. The trolley car problem pits the alternative as passive complicity with a greater number of deaths.

While most people would flip the switch, a more difficult variant places you on a bridge with the trolley hurtling down the track, under the bridge, and directly toward five people tied to the track. The only way to stop the trolley is to drop something very heavy from the bridge to land directly in front of the trolley. It so happens that there is a fat man standing nearby who is heavy enough to stop the trolley. Should you push him over to save five people? Most people have more trouble with this one and opt not to push the man over. Withholding food is passively allowing the death to occur. It is indirect, in a way, like flipping the switch. Administering barbiturates to cause death is more akin to pushing the man over the bridge. Our natural moral systems get easily discombobulated when pondering these dilemmas.

The use of brain imaging has provided entirely new insights into age-old moral dilemmas. By scanning individuals in a functional MRI while asking them to ponder the trolley car problem, Joshua Greene at Harvard University and Jonathan Cohen at Princeton University learned exactly which brain areas get engaged in solving the dilemma.[5] In essence, two brain regions come into play—one used for reasoning and the other for emotion. The rational part of the brain computes the fewer number of deaths and the emotional part of the brain contemplates the very high mental barrier we face in actually committing a murder. These stories are designed to bring the two brain regions into conflict.

Applying this simple dichotomy to the issue of prolonging life in advanced Alzheimer's disease, we might assume that decisions will be based on a similar balance of emotion and rationality. However, given identical circumstances, reasonable people can come to quite different conclusions. For example, how do we explain cases in which the family wants to stop all feedings, but the staff refuses? Certainly one would assume that family would have a greater emotional attachment to the patient and staff would be capable of a more detached, rational viewpoint. Real life does not pose the trolley car problem. A more likely explanation has to do with individual variation in how we make decisions. When families or staff differ over prolonging the life of an individual with advanced Alzheimer's disease, they must give different weights to the emotional and the rational sides of the argument. On the rational side of the equation, a discussion is possible. For example, the parties can lay out in detail why they do or do not want to withhold water as well as food to hasten death. They can provide evidence whether a person with advanced Alzheimer's disease would be uncomfortable because of excessive thirst—or whether the person's perception of thirst is completely blunted by the brain degeneration. However, when those whose opinions are based upon the rational argument encounter those whose decisions are mostly emotional, the same conflict that occurs inside the brain breaks free and can cause intense disagreements.

The emotional brain is a hub for angry outbursts, rage, and passion. Presenting the case for withholding life support to the emotional brain is not a matter of ticking off each reason—to the emotional brain, the sum of many reasons is no greater than any one alone. Each argument meets the same barrier. Consensus requires advancing one's point of view along two fronts simultaneously. Crossing the boundary, bringing an emotional or a rational argument to the other side, is useless because separate rules and separate thinking apply. What flies in one domain is doomed in the other and will more likely result in hostility. We watched these two brain regions play out their radically different bases for decision making on the national stage when in the predawn hours of March 21, 2005, President Bush signed into law an act for the relief of the parents of Theresa Marie Schiavo, which allowed her family to file suit in federal court in the hope that her life could be forcibly sustained.[6]

FACING THE PROSPECT OF ALZHEIMER'S DISEASE WHILE STILL COGNITIVELY INTACT

As we discussed earlier in this chapter, it is increasingly possible to predict whether a person will contract Alzheimer's disease. The accuracy of the prediction is very high in a few rare genetic cases and the accuracy of prediction is getting better in sporadic cases. Even without testing, some people, through introspection and tracking their own mental states, come to the conclusion that they are victims of Alzheimer' s disease. It is easy to worry that every time you forget where your car is in the parking garage you have just experienced the opening shot of Alzheimer's disease. But these common acts of forgetfulness do not suggest the disease. Some have said that Alzheimer's disease is not forgetting *what* you had for lunch, but that you *even had* lunch.

Suppose you find yourself concerned enough to undergo some testing and you learn that you are in the earliest stages of the disease. You are also very clear that you would prefer to die rather than live in need of total care. What are your options? One option is to prepare a directive that spells out your wishes in explicit detail. You might be sure that your family and your doctor know about this document. You might review your finances and decide the kind of care you can afford. You might attempt, over time, to have a series of discussions with family members about the burden they would have to assume in caring for you. All these considerations and discussions are emotionally taxing and challenging, and it is hard to anticipate every eventuality. You may want to assuage your fears, and the way to do so is to habituate yourself to the idea by thinking about death five minutes a day to be free of its terror. But the overarching issue still remains: taking one's life.

While this option might seem extreme and unusual, in fact, it might be neither. A few inferences from the medical literature suggest that a sizable number of elders have opted for suicide in the face of impending Alzheimer's disease. The statistics concerning suicide among the elderly are staggering. The National Strategy for Suicide Prevention Web site, which is sponsored by the Department of Health and Human Services, has collected the following data:[7]

- The highest suicide rate of any age group occurs among those sixty-five and older. Within this group the highest rate is for white males who kill themselves at a rate of 29 per 100,000 population.
- There is an average of one suicide among the elderly every ninety minutes.
- In 1998, suicide ranked as the sixteenth leading cause of death among those sixty-five and older and accounted for 5,803 deaths among this age group in the United States. Since that time the rate of suicide has varied very little in this age group.
- Suicide has a disproportionate impact on the elderly. In 1998, this group represented 13 percent of the population, but suffered 19 percent of all suicide deaths.
- The rate among adults from sixty-five to sixty-nine was 13.1 per 100,000 (all rates are per 100,000 population), the rate among those aged seventy to seventy-four was 15.2, and the rate for those aged seventy-five to seventy-nine was 17.6. For those in their eighties, or older, the rates continued to increase. Among those eighty to eighty-four, the rate was 22.9, and among people eighty-five or older, the rate was 21.0.
- Firearms (71 percent), overdose (liquids, pills, or gas, 11 percent), and suffocation (11 percent) were the three most common methods of suicide used by people aged sixty-five or older. In 1998, firearms were the most common method of suicide by both men and women, accounting for 78 percent of men and 35 percent of women who committed suicide in that age group.
- Risk factors for suicide among older people differ from those among the young. In addition to a higher prevalence of depres-

sion, elders are more socially isolated and more frequently use highly lethal methods. They also make fewer attempts per completed suicide, have a higher male-to-female ratio than other groups, have often visited a healthcare provider before their suicide, and have more physical illnesses.

- It is estimated that 20 percent of the elderly (over sixty-five) who commit suicide visited a physician within twenty-four hours of their act, 41 percent visited within a week of their suicide, and 75 percent have been seen by a physician within one month of their suicide.
- Suicide rates among the elderly are highest for those who are divorced or widowed. In 1998, among men seventy-five and older, the rate for divorced men was 3.4 times and widowed men was 2.6 times that for married men. In the same age group, the suicide rate for divorced women was 2.8 times and for widows 1.9 times the rate among married women.
- Several factors relative to those over sixty-five will play a role in future suicide rates among the elderly, including growth in the absolute and proportionate size of that population, health status, availability of services, and attitudes about aging and suicide.

These suicide statistics coincide with the Alzheimer statistics that also point to increasing risk with advanced age. Might the onset of Alzheimer's disease contribute to these suicides? A small but quite revealing study from Bordeaux, France, followed a group of 3,777 community-dwelling individuals aged sixty-five or older for fourteen years.[8] During this time, 350 subjects developed Alzheimer's disease, and they were compared to 350 matched controls who did not develop Alzheimer's disease. As early as twelve years before diagnosis, neuropsychological tests showed that the group destined to get Alzheimer's disease could be distinguished from the controls. The test the investigators used is called the Isaacs Set Test, which asks a person to name all the words she can think of within a certain category in fifteen seconds. Categories such as animals or all words beginning with the letter G might be part of the test. The number of words generated in fifteen seconds is the measure of the test. Another feature of those destined to get Alzheimer's disease is that they are more likely to be depressed seven to eight years before the diagnosis of Alzheimer's disease. Perhaps this observation points to a harbinger of suicide risk.

Suicide data in elders cannot be explained only by an increased risk of suicide among people destined to get Alzheimer's disease. While

Alzheimer's disease is more common in women, suicide among elders is highly skewed toward men. While the incidence of Alzheimer's is fairly uniform across the elder population, suicide incidence differs significantly by geographic region. The suicide rate in Nevada is nearly three times the national average. The state also ranks first in the nation by an even larger margin in the number of elder suicides. According to the Centers for Disease Control and Prevention, from 1999 to 2004, the suicide rate among people older than seventy-five in Nevada was 48 per 100,000, compared with a national average of 17 per 100,000. The second-highest-ranking state during the same time period and in the same age range was Wyoming, with a rate of 40 per 100,000. As we learn more about the relationship between one's social milieu and successful aging, these geographic differences will offer clues to researchers.

When researchers delve deeper into these numbers and try to understand why elders kill themselves more frequently in Nevada, the overriding answer is loneliness.[9] Although the exact cause and effect relationships are unknown, loneliness in the Nevada group is associated with absence of family nearby, gambling addiction, financial strain, or the desire for a final spree before ending their life. With isolation comes poor self-care and health problems. To address this problem, Senate Majority Leader Harry Reid, a Democrat from Nevada, introduced the Stop Senior Suicide Act on July 23, 2007. Reid's own father was a victim of suicide. (The bill was referred to committee and never became law.) Every one of these statistics has a story. A sixty-eight-year-old man, who has led a full and satisfying life, walks out into the New Hampshire woods and freezes to death. A woman, whose children have grown and given her grandchildren, accepts her terminal cancer and overdoses. Sometimes the prelude is more troubling, tagged with alcohol and depression. Maybe it's the feeling that with all that life has given us, something is still missing. In *The Sun Also Rises*, Ernest Hemingway wrote, "Nobody ever lives their life all the way up except bullfighters," and years later, on July 2, 1961, he committed suicide in Ketchum, Idaho.[10]

Alzheimer's is like no other disease. Measures that families take to learn the wishes of elderly parents on end-of-life decisions are often inadequate, and they do not address the long decline that the disease brings. Alzheimer's patients, even those in the early stages, are often not equipped mentally to decide to discontinue treatment. Much as the hospice movement revolutionized the way Americans—and the medical establishment—treat patients at the end stages of life, our approach with community-based cognitive shops that offer aid and counseling to

8

ALZHEIMER'S IN THE INFORMATION AGE

Knowledge, say you, is only the perception of the agreement or disagreement of our own ideas: but who knows what those ideas may be? Is there anything so extravagant as the imaginations of men's brains? Where is the head that has no chimeras in it? Or if there be a sober and wise man, what difference will there be, by your rules, between his knowledge and that of the most extravagant fancy in the world?
—JOHN LOCKE, *An Essay concerning Human Understanding*

THIRST FOR INFORMATION IN A SEA OF INFORMATION

Type "Alzheimer's" into the search box on Google and up come more than twenty-three million hits. But ask yourself this: among the bewildering barrage, is there a single gem of truth? It's clear that perusing all these sites won't help. Anyone spending one minute on each site, including the time for the site to load, working every hour of the day, would find that it would take nearly fifty years to review all the Alzheimer hits.

Yet, short of a cure, what patients with Alzheimer's want—perhaps more than anything else—is information. They want to know about the most promising research leads, about what they can expect as the disease progresses, about the experience of others who have dealt with

Alzheimer's disease, about comfort measures, about the genetic risk of family members, and about the effectiveness of treatments, both those that have been approved and those in the rumor mill.

Every time a new finding appears in the media, patients wonder whether the discovery will open the door to a therapy and how they might gain early access to these promising treatments. The hope that some little-known treatment, some neglected research, some unexplored crevice of knowledge can be tapped fuels the search for information. Answers are not easy to find. However, armed with reliable information, people can reduce their likelihood of developing Alzheimer's disease or, if already affected by cognitive impairment, they can slow its progression.

Given an incurable disease such as Alzheimer's, it becomes easy to prey upon people's desperation. And, not surprisingly, the search for medical information is itself a minefield of misinformation. How can anyone make sense of the vast repositories of false information, of the purported treatments, of the anecdotes and hearsay? More daunting than the veracity of the information is its sheer volume.

So how can we find out what we need to know? The first impulse: ask the doctor. We might call this the expert approach. We train physicians, license them, and then agree that they are a reliable source of information. Is that indeed the case? In the case of Alzheimer's disease, a field in which the knowledge landscape is changing with each new issue of the medical journals, few doctors are able to keep pace. Much of the needed information lies outside the expertise of most physicians—even specialists. Information about risk based on genetics is burgeoning; however, most doctors in practice today have not even been trained in the basic principles of genetics (see chapter 3 for an in-depth discussion of this topic). In general, even neurologists are often not well informed about the latest information. Only a small fraction of highly specialized neurologists, as well as some geriatricians, have adopted Alzheimer's disease and other neurodegenerative disorders, such as Parkinson's disease, as a specialty. The number of such specialists is far too small to reach the large number of elders with Alzheimer's disease and the even larger number of people at risk.

One of the most common types of medical encounters in the clinical setting is an all-too-brief doctor-patient interview, followed by a few laboratory tests, and finally a second equally brief meeting during which the physician blurts out his or her verdict. Even if Alzheimer's disease is an accurate diagnosis, delivering such grave news in a curt and hurried manner angers families. The patient leaves such an encounter frustrated, angry, and full of questions. The patient goes elsewhere, seeking second and third opinions, all of which multiplies the burden placed upon the medical system. I have heard these stories over and over.

However, the physician, whose busy practice is just barely staying afloat due to declining Medicare reimbursements, has opted for the most efficient way to discharge his or her responsibilities. Any effort beyond announcing the diagnosis and prescribing one or two of the currently approved medications for Alzheimer's disease is nonreimbursable and will back up a physician's waiting room. In fact, physicians would prefer not to have patients with Alzheimer's disease in their waiting rooms at all because their sometimes odd behavior might make other patients uncomfortable. The leap to the diagnosis of Alzheimer's disease with such certainty, based on just a few clinical indicators, unnecessarily stigmatizes the patient. A definitive diagnosis of Alzheimer's disease requires visualization of the characteristic brain pathology, the plaques and tangles. At the very least, it requires some sense of the clinical course of the disease to distinguish it from other dementias.

Here is another way to look at it. If a patient who is obviously demented comes in accompanied by a spouse, chances are good that the spouse already knows the nature of the problem. The physician might add the label, calling it Alzheimer's disease. However, a definitive diagnosis of Alzheimer's requires looking at brain tissue under the microscope. The physician may be able to help confirm or deny the presence of dementia, but once again he or she cannot know the disease is Alzheimer's. So why are physicians so quick to tell patients they have Alzheimer's disease when certainty in the clinical setting is nearly impossible? A realistic discussion that Alzheimer's disease is one possible explanation rather than an unrealistic pronouncement is more honest and less stigmatizing. Nevertheless, in strictly medical terms, the brusque physician usually does provide the correct diagnosis and the correct therapy. The physician has discharged his or her duty. But have the needs of the patient been met?

Once the diagnosis is made, the physician more or less says *adios* for the ten-year average interval between diagnosis and death. When the condition worsens, the physician has little to offer. Patients and their families embark upon an odyssey in search of information. The physician has not technically done anything wrong; he or she has simply exited the stage, leaving a dissatisfied patient and family in need of services that do not exist and information that is difficult to find.

A burgeoning number of online tools and health Web sites have come along to distill medical knowledge for family members and caretakers. In 2008, health Web sites attracted seventy-two million unique visitors, according to the online marketing research firm comScoreInc. That number represented a 14 percent increase from the previous year. According to the Pew Research Center's Internet & American Life Project, 60 percent of US adults turned to the Internet for health information in December 2008, up from 31 percent two years earlier. Among the services some of these health sites offer are entry of personal data that will trigger customized alerts and health messages. Among the most popular sites are WebMD Health Corp. and two other sites— Revolution Health and EveryDayHealth—that have recently merged. But these sites bombard users with advertisements every step of the way. Searching WebMD with the term "Alzheimer's disease" on January 8, 2009, gave a list of links that were a scattershot view of the subject, with no sense of a more fine-grained direction, no guideposts to pursue the answer to a question. At the top of the page under "Hot Topics in Alzheimer's Disease," the number one item was "Alzheimer's may be linked to overactive bladder." When you click on that link, you see advertisements for medications to control overactive bladder, but not a word on Alzheimer's disease. Although Alzheimer patients (as well as many other people) have an overactive bladder, this sort of linking does a disservice, funneling users away from top-level information. While these sites are not completely hijacked by advertisements, the presence of the advertisements diminishes users' confidence in them.

Some sites are moving our connection to online information forward. Consumermedsafety.org, sponsored by the nonprofit Institute for Safe Medication Practices, offers consumers approaches to learn about medication safety. The site allows users to enter the names of medications on an online form and the institute will send information on drug-safety ratings, possible interactions with other medications, side effects, and reviews from other patients. WhyNotTheBest.org from the nonprofit Commonwealth Fund evaluates and compares care at 4,500 US hospitals according to measures such as safety and good care. The site requires some medical sophistication because it provides specific data on good medical practice, such as giving aspirin to heart attack patients on arrival and preventive treatment for blood clots in surgical patients. The site uses data from Medicare's Hospital Compare Web site and the federal government's Hospital Consumer Assessment of Healthcare Providers and Systems survey. HazMap (hazmap.nlm.nih.gov) tracks information about exposure to potentially hazardous chemicals and biologics at work or by use in certain hobbies. This site can even be searched by job type for information about specific occupational hazards. Although Alzheimer's disease has not been linked to any toxin exposure, the question of toxin exposure comes up frequently in patient interviews.

With important information tucked away in the various corners of the Internet, we need to ask about use of the Internet among elders. According to the US Department of Commerce, the elderly are among the fastest growing groups of Internet users. As younger, more computer-savvy generations reach retirement age, Web use will only accelerate. Although estimates of Internet use are invariably out of date before they are published, one estimate claimed that 62 percent of Americans with Internet access have used it for medical information searches, and that six million are accessing health-related Web sites every day.[1] When older people use the Internet, it is more likely that they are seeking health-related information.

To that end, Web site designers and search engine developers need to keep in mind the cognitive and sensory changes that accompany aging. For example, macular degeneration may make certain fonts hard to read, trembling hands may make a mouse harder to control precisely, and an overly crowded Web display may distract or confuse when it is intended to provide information.

FROM INFORMATION TO KNOWLEDGE: SOCIAL NETWORKS AND THE MEDICAL WIKI

How do we know what we think we know? To narrow this long-standing epistemological question, let's focus on the realm of medicine. Two sources of knowledge exist regarding medical conditions. Expert knowledge is the kind acquired by those who read the primary scientific papers, examine findings from controlled studies, and, by virtue of their training and their advanced degrees, carry the weight of authority. The second is "wiki" knowledge, the kind that arises from collective experience. Today, the knowledge of the designated expert is increasingly challenged by the collective experience of ever-expanding cyber communities. We are undergoing a wikification of knowledge. This contemporary conflict represents a challenge for many disciplines that must balance expert views with those of the cyber community.

When medical findings are announced, whether they encompass a new therapy, a new preventive measure, or a new research finding, the patient cannot assume that the expert opinion of the physician is definitive. The limitations of the expert approach need to be clear. For example, let's consider treatment decisions with a newly approved med-ication for Alzheimer's disease. To get approved by the FDA, the phar-maceutical company had to prove safety and efficacy. But how fre-quently does the drug fail to work, and do other health-related factors such as lifestyle or coexisting disease or genetic risk affect the likelihood the drug will work? For example, evidence is emerging that some Alzheimer drugs undergoing clinical trials may have different thera-peutic effects depending on whether the patient has the Alzheimer risk gene APOE4 allele or not. Is there a way to find people predisposed to undesirable side effects? These are difficult questions for the expert. In the case of the most commonly used drug in Alzheimer's disease—donepezil—the physician has no idea about enhanced or diminished benefits in conjunction with other health factors and usually does not mention to the family that many users show no benefit at all.

Perhaps the power of the wiki could provide more depth for those making a decision about a drug treatment or a surgical procedure or the interpretation of a medical test result. So how can we create a wiki-based knowledge environment for medical information or make those existing sites more effective? In times past, collective knowledge derived from folk medicine, old wives tales, and anecdotal reports. The number of contrib-utors to collective knowledge in any one community was small, and the conclusions were clinically suspect. A small sample carries no statistical significance and can easily arrive at the wrong conclusion by chance. Nev-ertheless, anecdotal information—believing what your friends tell you—can have a powerful influence on people's decision making.

The modern-day version of folk medicine is no longer confined to a small circle of happenstance encounters within the limits of our physical geography. With the disappearance of geographic boundaries, links to medical conditions like our own can reach across the globe. Large num-bers of people—well beyond the numbers found in most medical studies—can build disease-oriented social networks with layers of added information and with an ease of follow-up to create a living, dynamic wiki. From the network, researchers can cluster individuals in any way desired—by geographic location, by occupation, by response to a medication—and patterns and correlations can be extracted.

How would a medical wiki work? An interest group in lifelong cog-nitive health would establish a site that combines the features of Wikipedia with those of Facebook. Wikipedia is a free Web "encyclo-pedia," open to everyone. At its best, it is a compendium of the wisdom of hundreds of thousands of users. At its worst, it allows people with a grudge or a particular bias to enter content that may not be objective or accurate. For example, a user could sign onto Wikipedia and enter information on President Obama that reflected personal opinion or repeated rumors. But because Wikipedia is open to anyone who wants to use it, the site has attracted a global following, and inaccurate or biased entries are often quickly corrected. The very term "wiki" means fast in the Hawaiian language, and wiki Web sites are now used widely at companies or by groups of people with common interests who want to communicate information quickly.

Facebook is an increasingly popular social networking Web site that allows users to register and create a Web page that includes a photo and biographical information. Facebook allows users to quickly create an online "community"—they can type in the name of a friend or colleague or even a celebrity, and send an e-mail request to include them on a list of friends. Facebook users can get automatic updates whenever another friend adds something to his or her Web page, and, in fact, that is part of the appeal. Users post photos of children and grandchildren and vacations, and paste in Web links to favorite articles and even videos. Use of Facebook has spread widely, beyond the original target audience of teens and college students. In fact, during the 2008 presidential campaign, news organizations like ABC created Facebook sites and posted interviews, videos, and debate commentary.

The user community would maintain the wiki portion of the site by distilling, commenting upon, and offering experience with the many potential remedies that keep the Alzheimer rumor mill churning. Does turmeric have any use in Alzheimer's disease? Should I drink green tea to prevent the disease? Does aluminum exposure cause Alzheimer's? At first, the experiences people post on the site would be haphazard and anecdotal, but as the site grows, the collective experience of many will become more valuable. The user community would be loosely overseen by a system that categorizes entries—for example, all entries on green tea would be collected and tabulated. If the topic gains interest, a questionnaire would be posted to the user community to obtain more structured information. As the results come in, they would be linked to any existing formal studies so as to put wiki knowledge and expert knowledge side by side.

As information accumulates on large numbers of people, it becomes possible to shuffle the data in any way one would like. How many people who drink green tea are also over age sixty-five? How does the blood pressure of green tea drinkers compare to that of those who do not drink green tea? If green tea drinkers tend to have lower blood pressure, then we can formulate the hypothesis that green tea might lower one's blood pressure. That hypothesis would then have to be tested more formally using a randomly selection of both green tea drinkers and those who do not drink green tea. The information deposited on the Web will always have the bias of being posted there by a select group. It is very possible that those who care enough to drink green tea and care enough to join a health-oriented social network take care of themselves in other ways, too, and therefore have lower blood pressure for reasons other than simply drinking green tea. Within social networks lies untapped wiki knowledge poised to challenge the experts by opening wide the collective knowledge gate. On a large enough scale, the collective experience of several million people begins to rival what can be learned from controlled studies by experts.

On the Facebook side, users would enter relevant medical information, a narrative description of their memory or thinking problems, and some biographical information, such as occupation, education level, family history, and geographic location. By checking a box next to each entry, the user would decide on the information that would be released to the network for viewing by other users. The user could set an allowable degree of separation for viewing personal data. One degree of separation from another person means that you know that person directly. Two degrees of separation means that you know a person only through the friends of your friend.

It is commonly claimed that all the world's population is connected by no more than six degrees of separation. Some people may be inclined to share personal medical information only with their close friends, while other people may be inclined to make their information more widely visible through the Web site. However, the real utility of this system is for the researcher to find pockets of good or bad health practices. A Webmaster compiles all the entries and strips out identity so members of the network can view the collective features of the network. Anyone can quickly see how many users are taking a particular supplement or a particular prescription medication, or see the range of blood pressures in the network, the geographic distribution of users, and the categories of occupations among users. As issues arise, users can turn the site for information and support. For example, a person who develops a symptom after taking a medication can alert the Web site and the Webmaster can issue a query to all users of that medication. Reporting through a social network has inherent drawbacks such difficulty in validating people's entries, but stacked against our current system of hodgepodge reporting, it offers valuable information and another early warning system to alert the people about adverse effects.

With this virtual structure in place, can social networks rival what is learned from expert approaches such as controlled studies and disease registries? Sound conclusions in the medical field are based upon statistical significance. The statistical power of a population, in other words, the ability to distinguish between an experimental and a control group for a particular research question, often depends on having a sufficiently large study group. The best way to increase the number of participating individuals is to tap into the Web. However, because of its open nature, the Internet is not a forum that lends itself to the well-controlled groups that researchers need for scientifically valid studies. On the other hand, the vast potential for touching enormous numbers of people could make the Internet a useful tool for some types of research. After all, researchers sometimes focus on extremely large groups of people in order to test a theory. Wiki knowledge derived from a social network offers a fluid, open-source, ongoing meta-analysis—a virtual collection of experiences that can be constantly updated as users enter more individual data.

Those we now deem as experts hold advanced degrees and have publication track records to support their claim to expertise. In the wikified environment, new breeds of experts will arise. A sense of their presence predates Web-based social networks. For example, among doctors in the community, some physicians are considered opinion leaders, and these are the people who will likely most influence Web-based decision making among users of social networks. How such people are anointed is partly based on their qualifications as traditional experts, but social science research reveals other factors that determine how we grant leadership status within social networks. The vehicle by which expertise can arise in virtual space comes through creating a well-functioning platform, such as on the highly researched Web site Alzforum (www.alz forum.org) founded by June Kinoshita. This site contains highly reliable information about Alzheimer's research managed by full-time science journalists, who consult frequently with primary researchers in the field. Input is allowed from users, but content is reviewed and highly controlled—not just anyone can upload a live post. In order to increase and expand the knowledge within social networks, Microsoft Live Search QnA (which has been released in a pilot version, known as a beta version) focuses on the emergence of expertise on a social networking site. The Microsoft site works like other social networking sites that let the public pose questions in a Web forum. Questions on Microsoft Live Search QnA are not specifically for doctors or patients. Instead, the site is an example of how the power of social networking could be harnessed for specialized topics like Alzheimer's. Questions are posed to the entire community of users. People who use the Microsoft site establish expertise by gaining points for how well they answer questions. The questions are posed to the entire community, not to a single expert. The user community votes on the quality of the answers provided and a high scorer emerges. Questions fall into topic areas. A user develops a good reputation by gaining the approval of the user community on several questions within a topic area. Presumably, this is a self-reinforcing process because once a user develops a good reputation, his or her future responses will have more influence. How this approach would operate in a medical setting is unexplored territory.

Social networks empower the expert—who could be a trained professional or an educated layperson with a knack for research—because access to this community-generated knowledge is shared by all. For example, at Love Canal, twenty-one thousand tons of chemical waste lay buried beneath the community unbeknownst to the residents. Back in 1978, a time long before social media existed, Lois Gibbs, a local mother and president of the Love Canal Homeowners' Association, first associated exposure to the leaking chemical waste with the epilepsy, asthma, and urinary tract infections that were recurring in her children. Although flagrant and clear cut, Love Canal is not unique. Now, the ability of Web-based medical networks to cluster data geographically has the potential to reveal other dangerous living conditions. Similarly, occupational risks for disease are well recognized, and organizing medical data in this way will likely serve as an early warning system for on-the-job risks. Existing information sources such as a keyword search on the Internet leave one smothered under a blanket of irrelevant information, and existing organizations such as the Alzheimer Association may not even be aware of emerging associations between disease risk and environmental factors.

Web-based medical networks represent an approach to what is now a completely intractable problem. How can one possibly capture multiple simultaneous variables when computing risk for Alzheimer's disease? Multiple simultaneous variables plague most medical studies. For example, does a study that reports a benefit or a risk for, say, memory impairment among coffee drinkers control for the number of hours those people spent in the gym? In this case, the researchers have to measure the degree of memory impairment, the amount of coffee, and the hours engaged in exercise. These are all called variables. When a new drug is tested, the control group may not be identical to the experimental group in caloric intake, number of portions of vegetables eaten, or amount of daily exercise. At best, the study is controlled for age and gender. But if those taking the drug are eating poorly and under stress and those on the placebo are dining on salads and jogging on the beach, potentially inaccurate conclusions could be reached. And if one adds the genetic variation found in human populations—certain types of genes can increase or diminish the risk for disease—the variables mount further.

Controlled studies are not empowered to capture multiple variables—and medical conditions are brimming with variables. The problem is that most medical interventions, particularly those related to lifestyle like diet and exercise, do not result in clear-cut, black-and-white results. Some people respond well, others do not respond at all, and most are in between. To learn whether improving diet or increasing one's exercise or a host of other remedies are effective requires testing them on large numbers of people, and the more remedies we test, the more people we need as subjects. Social networks are perfectly designed to gather the large number of subjects needed to reach more definitive conclusions.

Networked medical data will have an impact far beyond Alzheimer's prevention. It might at last break the refusal of surgeons to publish their outcomes. For many surgical procedures, outcomes are directly related to the experience of the surgeon, or how many times has the surgeon performed the operation now recommended for you. And what is his or her complication rate and success rate? Although that information is collected in many hospitals, patients are not allowed to see it even if they ask. A network that includes a set of patients all operated upon by a single surgeon would contain exactly that information. However, some notes of caution must be mentioned. If very few people report on a surgeon, the medical wiki data are skewed toward the few whose opinions may not be representative. Participation is important to make this work. We may look at a few random movie reviews on the Web before choosing a movie, but we are more likely to choose a movie that was liked by whose taste is similar to ours. And so Web-based opinions of surgeons might be tempered by an objective moderator. Nevertheless, statistics concerning complications and mortality speak for themselves. Another caveat is the disgruntled patient who wants to smear a surgeon and fabricates multiple entries with bad outcomes. Tools are needed for verification and space for the physician to provide a rebuttal.

A more complex public statistic involves quality measures that grade an entire hospital. A recent report on California hospitals found that they vary widely on mortality for eight common procedures, including hip fracture, carotid endarterectomy (a surgical procedure to remove fatty plaque from the carotid arteries in the neck), and brain surgery. Any major hospital procedure can affect one's cognition, especially in elders, and, therefore, knowing something about a hospital's performance is useful before an elective procedure. This information on hospitals has been posted at http://www.oshpd.ca.gov. But these data must be interpreted with caution because hospitals differ regarding the number of concomitant conditions, or comorbidity, their patients have—some hospitals are more likely to treat sicker patients or older patients or to discharge patients quickly before complications set in. Perhaps as important as the mortality figures are the number of cases in each category. Hospitals with a high volume of surgical procedures are likely to have one or two staff surgeons who perform most of the specialized surgeries.

While drugs are only a stopgap measure for Alzheimer's disease, there are implications for drug data as well in a networked system. Important data about the prescribing habits of physicians are also kept from patients, but could be included in a Web search. While the patient does not know which drugs his or her doctor prescribes, the drug representative sitting outside the office waiting to inform the physician about his company's products knows—exactly. Drug companies know the prescribing history of nearly every physician through data warehouses. Physicians are ranked nationally by volume of all prescriptions written for a particular drug.[2] Based on the rankings, physicians are labeled as "high share" users, meaning the physician uses a lot of one company's products, or "uncommitted splitters," meaning the physician splits his prescriptions among many products from different companies. Other terms are also used to describe physicians, such as "loyalists," who prescribe drugs made by a single pharmaceutical company; "sample-grabbers," which is self-explanatory; "hidden gems," who are considered susceptible to a marketing pitch by a drug sales representative; and "drug-whores," who switch loyalties among pharmaceutical companies. All this information is compiled by a few lucrative industries, the largest of which is IMS Health, located in Norwalk, Connecticut, with $2 billion in revenue in 2007. IMS Health and other similar companies buy a physician masterfile from the American Medical Association (AMA). The sale of the file is a major source of income to the AMA. Knowing the drugs physicians tend to prescribe is very revealing. If your physician is a "loyalist," you can pretty well guess which pharmaceutical company makes the drug you will be prescribed. While physicians deny they are influenced by marketing, the large sums of money poured into compiling dossiers on physician prescribing habits speak loudly against this view.

One of the overriding reasons that the social network wiki will have an impact on the problem of Alzheimer's disease is related to the startling recent insight discussed in chapter 3—Alzheimer's disease is not the most common cause of dementia in elders. Once in a community setting, rather than the highly selected patient groups studied by academics, the most common form of dementia is actually "mixed dementia." This term refers to Alzheimer's disease and vascular dementia, which frequently occur together. In the former, plaques and tangles are found on neurons; in the latter, the condition impairs brain blood flow. Because most dementia in the community is due to a mix of both Alzheimer's disease and vascular dementia, if these patients were treated with a drug that cured Alzheimer's disease, they might still have dementia because of the vascular component. The physician treats community-based dementia with the best available medications for Alzheimer's disease but pays scant attention to diseases of blood vessels. Expert knowledge derived from studies of people with pure Alzheimer's disease might not be applicable to the majority of people with dementia, yet we are basing nearly all our treatments on conclusions from groups of people with pure Alzheimer's disease. On the other hand, the collective experience of the community of dementia patients could more accurately reflect the nature of dementia among the majority of people. Within the community, the response of dementia to treatment might be more readily inferred from social networks of informed caregivers who cope with dementia on a daily basis.

Because the notion that medical knowledge can be gathered on a wiki Web site is unconventional, decisions based on a medical wiki need a dose of skepticism. A doctor could be swayed by an accumulation of anecdotes and draw conclusions based on a population sample that is not representative of the larger group. For example, those who participate in a social network tend to be younger and not economically disadvantaged. Older people will be less represented in Web-based data-gathering tools because they are not frequent users of the Internet. This barrier to comprehensive community-based information will bias any knowledge from this source. However, in time, the increasing penetration of the Internet to all segments of society will resolve this issue, as has happened for telephones and TV.

Through the network, unfiltered information bubbles up from a highly varied audience, and unanticipated knowledge can emerge. Social networks can be focused toward or linked to people with a specific disease or disease predisposition like Alzheimer's or vascular problems or rare forms of dementia. We know that, in exceptional cases, a patient with Lou Gehrig's disease (ALS) plateaus for many years, reaching a point at which the disease does not become worse, rather than suffering the inevitable decline of most patients. Sometimes, a patient with cancer spontaneously gets cured. No one has ever been known to recover from Alzheimer's disease—finding just one such patient would offer the potential for breakthrough scientific insights. Disease registries have been one approach to finding these outliers, but they are expensive and require time-consuming supervision at the top level. A social network may have a better chance to gather the number of people with relatively rare outcomes, determine what they have in common, and possibly learn why they beat the odds.

We know there is great variation in how people respond to drugs, but using population data rather than individual data loses many fine-grained features, such as how specific side effects may be associated with each other or what predicts who will benefit and who will fail. Among the currently available medications approved for Alzheimer's disease, there is great variation in how well people respond and whether they experience side effects. Social networks could contribute to learning the basis for the differences in drug response among individuals. Of course, the leveling effect of the Internet can displace the professional, who could be replaced by mass amateurism as people begin to self-diagnose and make their own medical decisions, perhaps sometimes due to their inability to afford a real-life physician encounter. No doubt there are obvious risks in this approach. On the other hand, Web-based data might reduce the frequency of mistakes made by medical professionals because decisions will be based on a very large-scale knowledge environment rather than what may be a highly skewed experience of a single physician.

The number of Web sites intended to create social networks centered on people who all share a disease is growing rapidly. Here is what might be called a tasting menu of such sites:

(1) dailystrength.org founded by Doug Hirsch. This site includes patients and caregivers dealing with hundreds of conditions, including Alzheimer's disease. The site includes support communities, wellness journals, personalized health information, advice sharing, doctor recommendations, and links to news stories and other Web sites including blogs, podcasts, customized search engines, and wikis in which users collaborate on Web-based information, such as with photo albums and contact lists, alerts to mobile phones and instant messaging, and even a virtual hug.

(2) Healia.com is a health search engine that ranks content on relevance and quality, including numerous hits on Alzheimer's information. Users add personal filters to find tailored health information.

(3) organizedwisdom.com covers many different medical conditions, including Alzheimer's, and has a newsy feel to it. When I accessed it on January 27, 2009, the lead story was Hilary Clinton's coughing attacks. The site has little health quizzes and personality tests.

THE PRIVACY ISSUE...OR NOT?

Some people worry a lot about privacy. Their worries range from concerns about identity theft to information leaks in the workplace that might damage their reputation to some nebulous sense that certain information needs to be kept guarded. While these concerns are legitimate, others hold that privacy is a nonissue. Where is middle ground? Where do we draw the line of reason and reasonableness on this contentious issue? Most people really don't care about other people's personal information, but a few have found a way to exploit this inherent weakness in electronic systems.

We delude ourselves by calling the problem one of privacy, however. More accurately, the issue is data protection. No network is totally secure—and medical information is not immune. Even more traditional medical records do not have completely secure privacy barriers. This past fall, staff at a Los Angeles hospital were discovered snooping through records of Hollywood celebrities. And this case is not unique.

Privacy, on the other hand, is something we may have too much of. The case has been well put by Jonathan Franzen in a *New Yorker* piece. Today, people are more private than they ever were in nineteenth-century small-town America. The anonymity of big cities affords more privacy than do small towns, where everybody seems to know everybody's business. The problem for many elders is not privacy, it is loneliness.[3]

Jonathan Franzen knows a thing or two about Alzheimer's disease as well. In his collection of essays, *How to Be Alone*, Franzen opens with "My Father's Brain," in which he reveals that a brain autopsy showed that his father had Alzheimer's. In the essay, Franzen artfully weaves in the history of the German doctor Alois Alzheimer, who treated fifty-one-year-old Auguste D., with his father's progression.

By the time my father's heart stopped, I'd been mourning him for years. And yet, when I consider his story, I wonder whether the various deaths can ever really be so separated, and whether memory and consciousness have such secure title, after all, to the seat of selfhood. I can't stop looking for meaning in the two years that followed his loss of his supposed "self," and I can't stop finding it.

Franzen normalizes the all-too-common experience of seeing an ailing parent through to the end, finding humor in some of it and meaning in most of it. It is as if Franzen is telling us: let us drop the veil of privacy and let the conversation begin.

Although information on the Internet is often viewed as having the potential for intruding on privacy, in fact, Internet connections hold the potential for rescuing homebound elders from their isolation, especially if we can overcome the barriers elders feel about going online. There is no doubt that online connections have quickened the pace of teenage social lives without jeopardy of privacy invasion. In fact, in the case of our own teenagers, we might wish for a bit less privacy in their constant texting. Certainly, the known benefits of friends and a social life on brain aging should be brought into the lives of elders as facilely as we have done for the young.

DOCTORS WILL NO LONGER DIAGNOSE

The shift of information resources to an easily accessible public realm will devalue the expert, and the physician is no exception to the rule. With so much information in the public realm and the smart tools needed to retrieve that information widely available, our tendency to turn to the doctor for a diagnosis of what ails us will diminish. The prevalent use of the Web to search for answers to medical questions is laying the groundwork for the public acceptance of medical diagnoses. The areas of cognition and memory function are well suited for online evaluation. But first some background.

Nearly from the time medicine became a discipline in its own right, the medical culture recognized the venerable expert, the professor whose opinion was considered authoritative, the final word. Historically, most of what the respected professor offered was diagnosis. In fact, most of what all doctors focused upon was diagnosis because most diseases could not be treated. Among diseases of various organs, treatment for afflictions of the brain has lagged behind because of the complexity of this vital organ and its inaccessibility. And treatment for Alzheimer's disease continues to lag.

When I began training as a neurologist, our discipline was known to exhibit a certain degree of "therapeutic nihilism." This derogatory term implied that neurologists were not particularly interested in treatment, and if they were, then they had little to offer. Raymond Adams, the chair of the department of neurology at the Massachusetts General Hospital from 1951 to 1977 and a giant in the field, is reputed to have said, "The reason people get neurological disease is so we can learn about the brain." This statement, which sounds harsh today, was perfectly reasonable in the context of its time because most neurological conditions had few, if any, treatment options. Among practitioners of that generation, few of the drugs we have today for epilepsy, migraine, Parkinson's disease, and multiple sclerosis were available. The majority of treatments for neurological conditions emerged in the past quarter century as neurologists have acquired a larger armamentarium to fight disease.

What distinguished a neurologist among other medical colleagues, especially at a time when treatment options were limited, was the ability to diagnose those cases that no one else could figure out or to surprise one's colleagues with a less obvious diagnosis when everyone else assumed the obvious. The distinguished neurologist was not only a master diagnostician but also performed his art with style and ease and often a bit of bravado. When I began my neurology training in 1977 at Tufts New England Medical Center, John E. Sullivan, a contemporary of Raymond Adams, had just stepped down as neurology chair. However, he continued to make occasional rounds with residents. A man of few words, he would walk into a patient's room and within moments tell us the correct diagnosis. Sullivan had that ability of the old-time masters to make an astute diagnosis on just a few, and not necessarily obvious, observations.

Over the ensuing decades, it has become possible to treat conditions that were previously intractable. For seizures we have gone from a single drug—Phenobarbital—to a mind-boggling number of different anticonvulsants. Likewise, for migraine, there are many drug options. Even strokes, if caught within the first few hours, are treatable. At the same time, diagnostic evaluations have become more automated and less reliant on the astute professor. The careful history and physical exam is slowly succumbing to the technical precision of instrumentation. Like neurologists who can now see the living brain with imaging technology, cardiologists rely on cardiograms and echocardiograms, while nephrologists turn to chemical analysis of the blood and urine.

Each field has developed its own incisive tools. When the medical student reveals the diagnosis by holding up an MRI or CT scan of the brain, even the professor has to acknowledge the indisputable authority of the technology. So neurology, with all its accompanying technological splendor, has become a less challenging discipline for diagnosis, and increasingly the role of the physician is to select and implement appropriate treatment.

The assessments used to evaluate memory and other cognitive functions when one is concerned about Alzheimer's disease are routine and in many cases can be conducted online as long as a caretaker is present to serve as an interface between the computer and the patient. Although somewhat counterintuitive, the greater the level of expertise and specialization, the easier it is to design an artificial intelligence system. The algorithms to reach a highly specialized neurological diagnosis are often well defined by established criteria. On the other hand, knowing whether to hospitalize a child who simply looks sick is hard to teach a computer, but it is a feat performed masterfully by the experienced pediatrician in general practice. Highly specialized knowledge is well suited for the Web because, like the Web, it is a growing and changing body of information that is easily kept current.

Obviously what is missing in this disembodied doctor-patient relationship is the human connection, the laying on of hands. As we increasingly dissociate medical knowledge, which is an Internet service, from the human warmth and connection of a truly satisfying and compassionate doctor, what model will work best? Perhaps the human connection in a medical encounter need not come from an expensive MD, who seems less and less equipped to provide the human connection anyhow. When health reform gets around to tackling the issue of cognitive health in elders, a setting such as the one described in chapter 2 creates a cost-effective program that balances more favorably the roles of various healthcare providers.

YOUR DOC GOES VIRTUAL

Increasingly, Internet communities may replace doctor-patient consultations. With the portability of images and other laboratory data now leading to remote offshore readouts, the doctor as diagnostician is becoming more irrelevant than ever. Dr. Amar Gupta, writing in the *Wall Street Journal* in October 2008, has described this offshore medical world. He points to offshore services such as the integration of health-information systems, drug-safety monitoring on a global scale, and more high-quality information gleaned from both expert sources and social networks to doctors and patients.

It may not seem palatable at first, but after awhile the ease and low cost of a virtual medical consultation may become preferable to seeing a physician. The impartiality and comprehensive depth of knowledge on the Web can exceed that of the individual physician and is more easily updated. Although the current state of medical information delivery on the Web has too many downsides to be a practical replacement for the physician, the trajectory toward increasing utilization of the Web in medicine is clear. We have already passed step one—the tendency of many people, maybe the majority of people, to consult the Web for their ailments before asking their physician. Medicine cannot buck the tidal wave of goods and services that are migrating to the Internet without any trace of a tangible physical presence or a real geographic location left behind.

To put e-medicine into the context of what is happening around us, just consider how much of our world even now lacks any physical presence. Business at retail stores is declining while Web-based retail is in the ascendancy; banking, bill paying, and taxes are all online, as are music, books, movies, and even many friendships. Whether aimlessly browsing (formerly known as shopping) or seeking a specific item, the Web has the appropriate search engine. Books, newspapers (especially their classified sections), and magazines are often more easily accessible on the Web than in the neighborhood. Nearly every piece of music ever recorded is downloadable, and movies are not far behind. Storing material versions of books and music is no longer necessary; they are more readily available on demand from the world of server farms and other means of distributed information. The sweeping changes of the online world become even more radical when they displace services. A large part of banking, airline ticket purchasing, travel planning, so-called adult entertainment, and higher education are already there. Gaining ground rapidly is the transfer of our social lives to the Web with social networking sites like Facebook, gaming communities, and ultimately a virtual existence in the form of an avatar on a site such as Second Life. Meeting people, dating, and long-term relationships can be conducted entirely *in silico*. So why not doctors?

The purveyors of information are improving their information delivery methods. Online sites offer medical information about searchable conditions and, indeed, provide a useful service. MedStory has added more intensive search tools that allow users to delve more deeply into a single topic. Typing in Alzheimer's disease, for example, produces a display of relevant topic areas that can be probed more deeply. Topic areas include drugs and procedures, in addition to personal health, complementary medicine, nutrition, and clinical studies. These later topics are not commonly addressed by physicians, but are frequently inquired about by patients. Unfortunately, the deeper level of the search leaves patients in the same quandary with too much undigested information. Some may not understand the material presented; others may find the shear quantity of information burdensome.

We need to know more about how people use these medical information sites, what kinds of questions they are posing, how often they get a satisfactory answer, and how often they get misled. The value of medical information will need to be assessed in terms of its accuracy, the adoption of the correct recommendations, confidence in the conclusions offered online, and the ever-present watchword of today—reduction of medical costs. No doubt having an actual person—not necessarily a doctor, but someone with medical sophistication—to talk to would help.

The Web is a rich source of information, but sorting and interpreting the facts remains a human task. Until artificial intelligence reaches the point at which the response from the computer is indistinguishable from that of a human being, having an actual person with the requisite medical knowledge somewhere in the mix will remain useful. To provide state-of-the-art information on cognition, a skilled professional, who serves as a human search engine, would be a useful link between patients and Web knowledge. The person guiding this kind of search is known as a Navigator. A human search engine uses input from other people in real time to filter results and help users clarify search requests.

The Navigator replaces one facet of what the physician does. Physicians have to answer the same questions over and over again. When dealing with Alzheimer's disease or most medical problems, for that matter, there is a standard set of questions that patients usually pose. Many of these questions can be handled by the Navigator. Although there are clearly a set of frequently asked questions among families of Alzheimer patients, the answers provided by the FAQ section on Web sites are usually inadequate and not sufficiently specific for the individual case. Among the questions often asked are those related to assisted living facilities, disagreements among family members about the best care management for their loved one, the risk that the disease may be passed to offspring, current research programs, and the value of various supplements. These are all topics in which physicians have little or no training, often have little interest, have too little time to address, and if they were to take the time to discuss these issues at length, they would not be reimbursed. In contrast, the Navigator is ideal for filling in information, particularly with the Internet at his or her fingertips so there is no need to create the illusion that the person providing the information is all-knowing. The Internet provides the Navigator with answers when the matter in question is changing rapidly, such as current clinical trials for treatments that are going on around the country and what criteria patients must meet to participate. Physicians do not generally know about trials in detail, but it is the type of data that can be easily displayed in a setting with a patient, his family, the Navigator, and a computer screen.

As a result, users receive a limited number of high-quality, highly relevant results instead of an overwhelming number of "hits," most of rather dubious value. Answers about genetic risk if a parent is affected or what is known about a recently reported healthy diet, or local resources for daycare are all fair game for the Navigator.

The human search engine or Navigator is not an MD. Simply put, the MD is too expensive for this position, is not trained in information retrieval, and is not particularly interested in some of the quasi-medical questions posed. A system that relies less on MDs and yet still provides state-of-the-art information will reduce medical costs. A single skilled Webmaster can keep a site updated with the latest research, in contrast to the enormous educational efforts required to keep an MD current.

This role does not remove the MD from the picture; it simply refines the doctor's job description by limiting a facet of the job that is now poorly performed. Our goal is to make the search sufficiently meaningful and productive so that we reduce the burden on physicians to supply information that may be only tangential to their specialty yet highly relevant to the daily life of the patient. Despite adding value to the services that physicians currently provide, MDs may not readily embrace the Navigator role. They may view Navigators as a threat to their practices, especially if the Navigator operation is established outside the physician practice where patients may be siphoned away. But, in fact, the Navigator will allow the physician to see more patients and focus on the medical issues. When patients collect Web-based information and present it to the physician, he often dismisses it without a glance. The reaction is arrogance of thinking that the patient can impart knowledge to the doctor rather than the usual doctor-to-patient information flow. Given the negative reaction of many physicians when presented with Web-based information, one might hope that physicians would appreciate someone who takes on the role of information gatherer and information validator.

The Navigator performs two main tasks: finding out what the person *wants* to know and finding out what the person *needs* to know. Need-to-know information is based on what experts in the areas of cognitive impairment have shown to be important. For example, designating power of attorney or the guidelines on driving privileges or attention to drug interactions may be important need-to-know pieces of information, depending on the stage of the disease. Want-to-know inquiries, such as information about supplements and new research discoveries, are cumulatively added to a list of frequently asked questions so the computer becomes smarter over time. Feedback from families is important throughout the process of searching for information. The Navigator, aided by a computer, can keep track of which answers prove to be the most useful and can use that history of successful searches to build a sort of directory. That directory can be used to point future users in the right direction.

Although having a live Navigator in the room is ideal, a remote Navigator could also be effective—for example, connecting through e-mail or instant messaging. The remote guide is the system of social searching adopted by ChaCha. Albeit not particularly directed toward medical questions, ChaCha is a site founded by Scott A. Jones, the inventor of voicemail systems. ChaCha uses human guides to assist in answering questions. According to its Web site, ChaCha becomes "smarter and faster" because it indexes questions with the search engines used by Guides (the humans performing the search) and the links visited by users. Feedback by patients or caregivers on the usefulness of some answer given by the user to the Guide influences the probability that the particular answer will be used again. In this manner, the search engine learns what information is relevant and useful for its users.

The Navigator has to be working with all available information. She needs to have all the necessary information about the patient in front of her so the computer can flag areas of medical concern. This information resource must be seamlessly integrated with personal medical data. But personal medical data is a confusing mishmash of entries by numerous physicians written in a cryptic manner, along with laboratory numbers and imaging reports (e.g., x-rays, CT scans, and MRI results). One way to think about personal medical data is to divide it into a narrative portion and a single-entry portion. The narrative is the person's story or medical history; the single-entry portion is made up of lab tests, prescriptions, and the like. One of the goals in moving toward an electronic medical record is to convert more and more of the narrative portion into a single-entry format. The patient's story is broken down with a series of questions that are answered with either yes or no. So instead of asking, "What first brought the memory problem to your attention?" the doctor might lay out a series of possible scenarios—Did you forget an appointment? Did you forget to pay your bills?—all with simple yes or no answers. Of course, much of the nuance of the narrative is lost with a single-entry format. And we all probably agree that losing the unique stories of our patients would further dehumanize the medical relationship.

However, by deconstructing medical systems into data acquisition and the more narrative facet of medical history taking we can improve the organization of our care delivery. Data acquisition is a by-the-numbers decision tree that requires a very different approach than listening to and responding to the often heart-wrenching stories we hear from our patients. Both are vitally important! Often the doctor draws a strictly-by-the-book conclusion from a set of bulleted patient data points. These types of conclusions will emerge from the single-entry data sets, and these conclusions are a good starting point when healthcare professionals begin to consider the individual circumstances of their patients. Sometimes the conclusions have to be modified when the unique story of the individual in front of us is being considered. But let's first consider the assessment of patients by single-entry data points.

Some of the most objective single-entry data points do not come from the doctor's office; they do not come from the traditional means of evaluation by family history or physical exam. Instead, they come from the laboratory, the imaging center, and the pharmacy. Having that data alone online and readily accessible when a patient or caregiver is posing questions to a Web site or to a Navigator would very much enrich the information that could be obtained. Some systems, such as Google Health and Microsoft Health Vault and others, are moving toward handling this kind of information. A direct conduit between the pharmacy and the Navigator that provides a list of medications, including their dosage, would greatly aid in crafting an effective medical approach. What is missing, but changing rapidly, is a seamless flow of information between the health record sites and the pharmacies and laboratories.

The personal medical record could be even more informative if the patient could easily provide some of the simple single-entry responses that are generated in the doctor's office, such as weight, heart rate, and blood pressure. This is becoming possible with devices such as the Intel Health Guide approved by the US Food and Drug Administration in July 2008. This eight-pound, in-home gadget that fuses technology and healthcare with a 40 gigabyte hard drive can be hooked up to wired or

wireless monitors of glucose, blood pressure, weigh scales, pulse oxime-
ters, or peak flow meters, and then make these data available for remote
Web-based interactions. The data are visualized on a touch screen and
the encrypted information is sent to a remote database when the device
is connected to the Internet via broadband. Microsoft programs claim
to be able to link to these devices and enter the information into medical records. Of course, the accuracy of these systems requires further
validation, but they offer the potential to revolutionize the current exor-
bitant care requirements of elders.

As one collects personal data on cognition, it may be useful to have a
baseline neuropsychological assessment. We are aided by having on
file a baseline cardiogram or blood test values because being able to compare two test results and detect a change is more important than having
only a single result. A single determination of the controversial test for
prostate cancer called PSA (prostate-specific antigen) is much less useful
than discovering an increase in the level over time. Likewise, having a
baseline determination of one's cognitive function through a neuropsychological assessment provides a baseline to detect future change.

The neuropsychological assessment is a brain fitness test. As is true
with weight and blood pressure, it is probably a good idea to know the
results of this sort of cognitive test. Such testing is a relatively sensitive
diagnostic tool for Alzheimer's disease and is reasonably successful at
distinguishing Alzheimer's disease from other cognitive disorders. Testing
can measure various symptoms that are being experienced by the patient,
such as depression, suicidal ideation, personality disorders, and other
psychiatric conditions. While it is very difficult to diagnose mild cognitive impairment with a single neuropsychological measurement, noticing
a decline in performance compared to a previously established baseline
level of cognitive ability is worrisome. Having this baseline measurement
is a good reference if one becomes concerned—and sooner or later just
about everybody becomes concerned about his or her memory. Recently,
the Alzheimer's Foundation of America in New York City released a
report advocating for widespread cognitive screenings after the age of
sixty-five or as early as fifty-five if genetic risk factors are present.

I recall a former neighborhood of mine where most of my immediate neighbors were in their sixties, seventies, or beyond. After I moved
in and word got around about my interest in Alzheimer's disease, nearly
every neighbor over a yearlong period asked to visit so I could spend a
few moments with them over the kitchen table and listen to their concerns about memory. Most of these visitors quietly requested that I
conceal their concern and their visit from their spouse. While these visits

were not an official medical encounter, an experienced neurologist can get a fairly good idea about a person's mental status in a simple conversation with a few stealth questions intended to probe the person's memory and thinking. These questions appear as routine chitchat and simply inquire about what one did that day or one's opinions about some news events. Of course, not everybody has the opportunity to chat with a neurologist over the kitchen table.

The only alternatives are making an appointment with a neurologist or online neuropsychological testing. What is available? Remember, neuropsychologists use a battery of tests that have been validated and standardized. These are paper-and-pencil tests often administered by a student and take a minimum of two to three hours to complete. Quickie tests—even those backed by a doctor's endorsement—cannot pretend to offer anything close to a genuine and informative neuropsychological assessment that includes the human element. The Web is full of quickie tests that lack real value and are therefore meaningless. But this shortcoming is changing.

Tests from OptumHealth Behavioral Solutions demonstrate much higher standards and are intended to provide clinicians with a Web-based assessment that measures general cognition. The forty-minute assessment is based on well-known and validated tests of memory; attention, executive function, and response speed; and mood, social skills, and emotional resilience. The United States is undertaking baseline cognitive screening of troops before deployment, and the broader application of these testing formats may be helpful for Alzheimer screening. Pharmaceutical companies are developing large-scale, fully automated cognitive assessments for clinical trials, and these formats too are likely to have broad applicability.

We should consider what is to be done with online neuropsychological test results. How can we be assured that the results will not be misused by others? In reviewing this entire area, Alvaro Fernandez, who writes the SharpBrains blog,[4] points out these key considerations, all of which serve as excellent starting points:

1. Make sure the test measures what it is supposed to, and with high degrees of reliability.
2. Have clear policies in place as to who can access which data and for which purpose.
3. Consider how and when assessments will lead to actionable personalized recommendations to improve or maintain cognitive functions. (In other words, at what point will a test result generate a recommendation for a treatment.)

So whether you are concerned about your memory or perhaps even over a broader range of medical issues, prepare for your doctor to go virtual. As this happens, the necessary healthcare savvy will increasingly fall squarely on our own shoulders. Even now, going into a medical setting armed with medical knowledge can prevent errors of both omission and commission on the part of the medical system. Comparing one's symptoms to a Web-based differential diagnosis and attempting to make a layperson diagnosis is increasingly common, but this is only the first step. Once Web-based diagnosis is enhanced by online neuropsychological testing, and perhaps other remote measurements, the already vanishing doctor will disappear further into the ether. Medical expertise will be available, but much of it will be remote. The absolutely essential human touch will require a different venue.

TELLING OUR STORY IN AN E-WORLD SETTING

As we move more into a world of online information shaped by single data points, like blood pressure and cholesterol values, we must not forget that a very big part of what patients want is a chance to tell their story. They want to describe the details of their situation. They want to tell someone about a seemingly trivial incident that angered them or made them happy. Most of this material has very little to do with reaching an objective diagnosis and developing a treatment plan. But without the opportunity to tell one's story, to tell the day-to-day trials of caring for an Alzheimer patient, the detached issuance of a mobile phone alert in a synthetic voice may not be heeded. In *How to Be Alone*, Jonathan Franzen writes, "This was his disease. It was also, you could argue, his story. But you have to let me tell it."

Following a therapeutic program requires building trust between medical personnel and the family. And trust is built from listening to people's stories and showing empathy. As we have noted, our expectation that doctors can assume this role is receding rapidly. Even if the doctor is willing to listen, he or she cannot usually afford to take the time to do so.

Anne Harrington, professor of the history of science at Harvard University, has presented an important, often overlooked facet of this issue. As she has written in her book *The Cure Within*, narratives have helped us to make sense of illness and suffering. These narratives have become rooted within our cultural histories and serve "to narrate our way out of the darkness." According to Harrington, narratives about faith, healing, stress, and many other "remedies" play a big part in our turning to religion, to healers of all stripes, and to support groups and stress counselors for relief from suffering.[5] In all of these cases, we buy into a mind-body relationship that we believe can affect disease. From the 1950s on, stress has been associated with each of the major diseases that has come into public consciousness. Harrington notes the attention to stress and heart disease after President Eisenhower's cardiac crisis. Later in the work of David Spiegel, a psychiatrist at Stanford University, stress was impugned in cancer. And now stress as a contributory factor for the great specter of our time—Alzheimer's disease—is gaining traction among researchers.

Fiction encompasses all of human experience—or as much as we can stand to write—and so disease inevitably works its way in. Illness becomes a cultural vessel, a metaphor on the stage, in fiction, and in the movies. So what begins as taboo becomes easier to approach. Art may afford just enough distance to allow us to apprehend. French philosopher Michel Foucault, who wrote about illness, the human body, and the place of medicine and science in society, observed that disease holds a place in many historical epochs: "Linked as they are with the conditions of existence and with the way of life of individuals, diseases vary from one period and one place to another. In the Middle Ages, at a time of war and famine, the sick were subject to fear and exhaustion (apoplexy, hectic fever); but in the sixteenth and seventeenth centuries, a period of relaxation of the feeling for one's country and of the obligations that such a feeling involves, egotism returned, and lust and gluttony became more widespread."[6]

Tuberculosis was the subject of Thomas Mann's masterpiece, *The Magic Mountain*, first published in 1924. Mann's sanitarium was a microcosm of irrationality and sickness, which critics have taken as a metaphor for Europe. The protagonist, Hans Castorp, comes to a world of eros and ideas through his feverish encounters.[7] Anyone growing up in the late 1940s and early 1950s remembers not only the Communist Red Scare but also the polio scare. Mingling in crowds or swimming at the municipal pool were forbidden; every child in elementary school knew someone who had been suntanned and vibrant one minute, diving off the high board, and then stricken and weakened by poliomyelitis. Everyone knew someone who returned from summer vacation fitted with a leg brace or, worse, someone who could not come back at all but rested in a wheezing iron lung in a clinic. In the 1980s, the human immunodeficiency virus (HIV) surfaced in the gay community, killing healthy young men and touching off a race among researchers to find a cure. AIDS took its place in the public eye, and became the subject of plays (*Angels in America*), movies (*Philadelphia*), and narrative non-fiction (*And the Band Played On*).

The medical profession itself is treated as a narrative by most—its data are amassed scientifically, but the adoption of the larger story sketched by the data depends on how the results of scientific studies are presented for the public. Because biomedical science is grounded in firm scientific principles, often we can actually explain how a person got a disease. For example, he contracted AIDS by having sex with a person infected by the AIDS virus, or she got breast cancer from the mutant gene she inherited from her mother. But science is unable to answer the "why question"—why did this happen to me? The more traditional role of the doctor as health adviser allowed him time to talk about the "why question," not strictly in the role of a physician, but in the role of one who offers comfort. Electronic medicine will further restrict the already shrinking time spent on the "why question" by physicians. Any treatment model that takes medicine online must be prepared to offer a vehicle for patient narratives. People need to tell their story, and it is as much a part of medicine as the pills we prescribe.

NOTES

1. D. P. Lorence and L. Greenberg, "The Zeitgeist of Online Health Search: Implications for a Consumer-Centric Health System," *Journal of General Internal Medicine* 21, no. 2 (February 2006): 134–39.

2. Stephen L. Hauser and S. Claiborne Johnston, "Scripts for Science: A New Wrinkle on Academic Ties with Industry," *Annals of Neurology*, pp. A13–A15, Published Online: November 7, 2008.

3. Jonathan Franzen, "Imperial Bedroom: The Real Problem with Privacy? We Have Too Much of It," American Notes, *New Yorker*, October 12, 1998, p. 48.

4. Alvaro Fernandez, http://www.sharpbrains.com/blog.

5. Anne Harrington, *The Cure Within* (New York: Norton, 2008), p. 126.

6. Michel Foucault, *The Birth of the Clinic* (New York: Vintage Books, 1994), p. 33.

7. Thomas Mann, *The Magic Mountain* (New York: Vintage, 1996).

9

THE CHALLENGE OF OPTIMIZING LIFESTYLES

Chief Justice: Do you set down your name in the scroll of youth, that are written down old with all the characters of age? Have you not a moist eye? a dry hand? a yellow cheek? a white beard? a decreasing leg? an increasing belly? is not your voice broken? your wind short? your chin double? your wit single? and every part about you blasted with antiquity? and will you yet call yourself young? Fie, fie, fie, Sir John!

Falstaff: My lord, I was born about three of the clock in the afternoon, with a white head and something a round belly. For my voice, I have lost it with halloing and singing of anthems. To approve my youth further, I will not: the truth is, I am only old in judgment and understanding.

WILLIAM SHAKESPEARE'S *HENRY IV*, PART II, ACT I, SCENE 2

We open this chapter with a caveat about a well-worn word— *lifestyle*—and about lessons that can be drawn from the irrational exuberance that creates its own bubble of expectations. Both call for a critical evaluation. A large number of lifestyles have been assessed for a possible benefit on cognition in elders. Boiled down to the essence, a beneficial lifestyle includes physical exercise, a healthy diet, the mental stimulation that comes from ongoing cognitive challenges, avoidance of chronic stress, and a circle of friends. These are the themes that surface repeatedly in the literature. Following a healthy path is a matter of habits, and habits take time to acquire and more time to alter. Those habits that increase the risk of Alzheimer's disease may seem harmless for many years, but the lifestyle decisions you make today will affect your later years.

The studies to test the efficiency of lifestyle interventions may ask whether they can boost thinking and memory skills in a healthy person, whether they can boost the cognitive functioning of someone with Alzheimer's disease, and whether they can prevent Alzheimer's disease. These are all important and related questions because prevention depends upon understanding risk factors and how we can protect against them.

Well-controlled studies in this area are difficult, so confusion over contradictory findings is frequent from one study to another, especially when researchers publish papers that are far from definitive. There are many papers in this field based on poorly conducted studies that fail in their efforts to draw strong scientific conclusions. The usually positive results reported in poorly conducted studies might be attributed to *irrational exuberance*, a term often attributed to former Federal Reserve chairman Alan Greenspan but actually coined by the economist Robert J. Shiller. His book by that title describes the "feedback loop theory of investor bubbles." According to this theory, when many people in the market begin telling others about the success of their investments, others rush in because they are lured by the promise of high returns. This group of hopeful investors forms a sort of social network, sharing information and news, often through word of mouth.

The same effect can be seen in medical research. Some Alzheimer professionals have concluded that quality studies strongly suggest that lifestyle interventions can improve or sustain cognition in elders. William Thies, the vice president of Medical and Scientific Relations for the Alzheimer's Association said, "We may not be able to do anything about aging, genetics, or family history, but research shows us that there are lifestyle decisions we all can make to keep our brains healthier as we age, and that also may lower our risk of developing Alzheimer's disease."[1] Based on this conclusion, then, we will discuss the even more challenging problem of implementing beneficial behavioral changes and adhering to a healthy lifestyle.

EXERCISE

Perhaps the strongest case for an intervention that affects the likelihood of getting Alzheimer's disease is exercise. Numerous well-performed studies have unequivocally concluded that physical exercise can reduce the incidence of cardiovascular disease, which is associated with impaired cognition, and few studies have linked exercise to lifelong cognitive health. Large, long-term collections of health data are particularly informative, and can be mined for trends that can then be tested in rigorous, scientifically controlled studies. The most definitive long-term study to assess disease risk factors conducted to date on older women's health is the Nurses' Health Study, which has followed 121,700 female registered nurses since 1976.[2] Over a two-year period, the Nurses' Health Study reported that higher levels of physical activity were associated with improved cognitive scores in 18,766 women. A similar study in men reported that those who walk at least two miles a day are 1.8 times less likely than sedentary men to develop dementia over a follow-up period of six years.[3] Two other prospective studies came to the same conclusion, demonstrating that exercise is beneficial even when begun late in life.

Another approach is to compare many studies for similarities and differences. One such analysis compared thirty-six physical activity studies in older adults and came to the same conclusion.[4] The more exercise one gets, the lower one's chances of contracting Alzheimer's.

These types of studies are called epidemiologic because they study populations in the community, and the best of them are called prospective because they first define a study population and then follow it. Done in this manner, a certain amount of bias is avoided that otherwise could arise from looking backward, or retrospectively, and finding what we want to find. In other words, if you ask people how much they have exercised in the past year, your findings will be less accurate than if you first select a group of people and then follow prospectively how much they exercise. Once the investigators have some epidemiological data in hand, next comes a randomized trial. In this case, people are randomly assigned to either an exercise group and a nonexercise group for some time period and then the groups are compared with regard to their memory and other cognitive function tests. In 2008, researchers in Perth, Australia, recruited volunteers who reported memory problems but could not be classified as having dementia. One hundred seventy participants were randomly assigned either to a group receiving some general information about good health practices and their usual care or to a home-based program of physical activity for just twenty minutes per day. One hundred thirty-eight participants completed six months of usual care or physical activity and then eighteen months later were assessed using the most widely used neuropsychological instrument, known as the Alzheimer Disease Assessment Scale-Cognitive Subscale (ADAS-Cog). This test provides fairly reliable measurements of one's cognitive function.

In this study, the researchers observed less cognitive decline in the exercise group, and the benefit was sustained over an eighteen-month follow-up period. Although the effect of exercise at home on test scores was modest, it was greater than any drug for preventing cognitive decline and progression to dementia in older adults with mild cognitive impairment. The shorter-term boost was comparable to that of donepezil, the most commonly used treatment for Alzheimer's disease. To the credit of these investigators, they interpreted their study quite conservatively: The study was only designed to check for the rate of decline among those with memory complaints, not the likelihood of actually getting dementia. As the researchers put it, "The effect size of the intervention [exercise] was small and, while it supports the concept that physical activity can reduce the rate of cognitive decline, the clinical significance of our findings remains to be established. Finally, the results of this trial cannot be used to infer that physical activity reduces the risk of dementia among at risk older adults, because the study was not [designed] to investigate development of dementia."[5]

Although the study of physical activity and cognitive decline showed only a small effect, there is overwhelming evidence that being physically active confers many other benefits. Yet 74 percent of adults in the United States do not meet the recommended guideline of at least thirty minutes of moderate-intensity physical activity on most days of the week. One impediment to regular exercise is the common view among the sedentary that working out an hour a day is overly self-indulgent and those who exercise are more devoted to their physiques than to their jobs or their families. However, a clear consensus now holds that, in addition to having a preventive effect on Alzheimer's disease, exercise provides a short-term boost to one's cognitive powers and can reduce depression and anxiety.

The beneficial effects of exercise begin in children. A 2005 study in the *Journal of Exercise Physiology* reviewed the performance of 884,715 fifth-, seventh-, and ninth-graders on a state-mandated fitness test in California and compared the scores to the reading and math performance of the same students on a standardized achievement test. The fittest students had the best test scores. The relationship was more obvious among those who engaged in aerobic fitness—exercise like walking, bicycling, or swimming that benefits the circulatory system. Exercises that increase muscle strength (e.g., lifting weights) or flexibility (e.g., yoga) were unrelated to academic achievement. Even naysayers of exercise must concede that an increase in the amount of time spent on physical health–based activities is not accompanied by a decline in academic performance. Flying in the face of the scientific evidence, exercise programs in schools are being cut and children are growing increasingly sedentary and unfit. These lifestyles increasingly adopted by our children will lead to an earlier onset of chronic diseases such as type II diabetes, obesity, and cardiovascular disease. Compounding the problem, these factors increase the risk for Alzheimer's disease, and given the lifestyles of many children, we can expect that they will be more likely to get Alzheimer's disease when they reach their sixth decade. Embedding the habit of regular exercise at an early age could deliver a large windfall for children.

We can get important insights by taking advantage of the shared biology between humans and other animals. The link between physical activity and improved brain function is also observed in animal data. Housing rats or mice in environments with running wheels increases the growth of neurons in those brain regions that are involved in learning and memory. Similar growth effects can be demonstrated using neuroimaging techniques in humans. In humans, physical training boosts different cognitive processes, especially functions that are known as executive control: scheduling, planning, working memory, multitasking, and dealing with ambiguity.[6]

These effects of physical activity fit well with brain imaging observations. Higher levels of fitness—and even improvements in fitness—were related to changes in the brain. One type of brain change that scientists look for is a change in the size of some part of the brain. The brain is not simply a homogenous slab of gelatin, although its nondescript gray appearance does look rather unassuming. Rather, the brain has numerous anatomical regions for different functions, such as language and memory and vision. One or more of these regions can grow or shrink while the rest of the brain does not change very much. With exercise, among those areas that enlarge are the temporal region, which is involved in memory, and the prefrontal region, which is involved in strategic planning. Strategic planning does not refer to picking a stock portfolio. Instead, it involves the nearly unconscious sequence of events we need to carry out to accomplish nearly any task. If you are told the cost of an item at the checkout counter, you have to know in which pocket you need to reach to find your wallet, plan which size bill you will use to pay for the item, get the change, and put coins back in one place and maybe the bills back in the wallet. All these events need to occur in the correct sequence. This is the job of the prefrontal brain, a region that is also vulnerable to Alzheimer's disease and accounts for much of the confusion patients experience when they attempt to perform everyday events. The size of these regions is often predictive of how well an older person performs. Aerobic fitness training also has measurable effects on tests like the functional MRI (fMRI), which does not measure the size of different brain regions, but instead measures how actively a brain region responds to a problem. The fMRI indicates how much energy a particular brain region is using to perform a task. If you are holding a king and a seven in blackjack, you have to decide whether to take another card or hold. Certain parts of the brain when faced with this decision use more energy than during a rest state and get activated. Older adults who walked regularly over a six-month period had increased activation in some brain regions; however, not the same regions as the black jack players. Other regions, involved in thought processes, called the middle frontal gyrus and superior parietal cortex, were activated. With exercise some regions of the brain—for example, one place called the anterior cingulate cortex—had less activation compared to a control group that simply did nonaerobic toning and stretching. This finding may seem paradoxical and even detrimental, but, in fact, when the brain functions well and becomes more skilled in a task, its energy use goes down. For example, learning Tetris requires lots of brain energy, but a skilled player uses much less brain energy. If a person is more challenged in performing a task, he made use more brain energy and activate a larger area of brain. In the very earliest stages of Alzheimer's disease people have to use more brain energy to accomplish the same goal as a normal person. Many of the brain regions affected by exercise are also targeted by age-related deterioration.

Another brain region that showed increased blood volume in exercising humans is a set of brain cells called the dendate gyrus, which reside in a seahorse-shaped structure called the hippocampus (which, in fact, means seahorse in Greek) and is critical for laying down new memories. The dentate gyrus is especially interesting because it is one of the few brain regions able to make new brain cells throughout one's lifespan. In contrast to many organs in the body that have turnover in their cells, most of our brain cells have to last a lifetime—they do not turnover. However, there a few brain niches where new cells are made throughout the human lifespan, and the hippocampus is one such place. Some scientists believe that once these new cells are born in the hippocampus, they travel to nearby brain regions and contribute to replenishing our memory abilities. At Columbia University Medical Center, a small group of middle-aged subjects took part in a three-month fitness training study. The increased blood volume they observed in the region of the dentate gyrus was exactly the pattern previously observed in mice that are actively making new brain cells.

So it seems likely that exercise will increase the proliferation and the survival of brain cells, especially in the memory area of the brain, the hippocampus. Data of this sort are strongly supported in many animal studies. Because brain cells are lost in the hippocampus in Alzheimer's disease, this natural cell replacement effect may be one of the bases for the observed benefits of exercise. Having shown that there are physical consequences for the brain when we exercise, the next step is to discover the specific brain molecules and genes that are locally activated during exercise. We are in the early days of this research and, indeed, some brain proteins have been associated with the effects of exercise. It's probably no surprise that taking a pill to induce these proteins and the effects of exercise, rather than actually doing a vigorous aerobic workout, is not yet on the horizon. So hold on to your gym membership.

Arthur Kramer, a University of Illinois psychology professor who has published widely in this field, has pointed out that exercise produces significant improvements in short-term memory. Aerobic exercise appears to be particularly effective in enhancing intellect—a benefit that starts immediately after the workout and continues for days or even weeks. Kramer, who directs the Biomedical Imaging Center at the University of Illinois, has had elders undergo magnetic resonance imaging (MRI) scans before and after six months of aerobic exercise. He has been quoted as saying that exercise produces patterns of brain activity of the sort typically seen in twenty-year-olds.[7]

The cognitive effects of exercise can even begin during the workout. In my case, jogging is one of the best times to ponder a problem or let my mind wander. Either way, ideas seem to surface. The only distraction is the need sometimes to write down these thoughts. I wonder whether watching TV or listening to an iPod while on a treadmill or a stationary bike suppresses the freedom of thought one might experience during exercise by locking the mind onto some external stimulus.

With the exercise link to cognitive health now quite conclusive, the next questions loom large. What are the best types of exercise—and how long and how often? At what point, if any, does excessive exercise become harmful? Is weight training also beneficial for cognition? Is it ever too late to start an exercise program? What medical conditions or medications might mandate some caution about exercise? Perhaps the most important question is how to motivate people to exercise, a topic we will treat below.

DIET

Evidence has accumulated that diet can affect the likelihood of getting Alzheimer's disease. But a problem remains: none of the studies on diet are randomized, a key part of scientific inquiry, and so do not have the same level of credibility as the studies that measure the effects of exercise. Unless the subjects in a medical study are randomly put into the special diet group or the no-diet group rather than selected to be in a special group for study, the conclusions do not have the same scientific validity as the conclusions on exercise. The diet that has gotten the most attention is the Mediterranean diet because researchers at Columbia University Medical Center found that it can lower the risk for Alzheimer's disease. The underlying idea behind the study was that a whole pattern of diet, rather than a single food, will affect Alzheimer's disease risk. This study, called a case-control study, is based on a group of people in New York City.[8]

A Mediterranean diet was selected because evidence already exists that the diet decreases cardiovascular disease, several forms of cancer, and the overall death rate. The group under study consisted of 2,258 people in New York City who did not have dementia. They were evaluated every 1.5 years for adherence to the diet, measured on a ten-point scale. The essential components of the diet are thought to be monounsaturated fatty acids, such as those found in fish oil, cereals, and wine. Adjustments were made for age, sex, ethnicity, education, caloric intake, smoking, genetic risk for Alzheimer's disease, and body mass index. The investigators concluded that a higher level of adherence to the Mediterranean diet was associated with a reduction in the incidence of Alzheimer's disease. Although this is a provocative finding, the study does not address the basis for how diet can affect the risk of getting Alzheimer's disease. In their next study, the same investigators reported that combining a Mediterranean diet with exercise reduced the risk of getting Alzheimer's disease more than either factor alone.[9]

We are a highly diverse lot in our tastes, so someone who can provide some personalized nutritional guidance can be invaluable in adopting a healthy diet. Dr. John LaPuma has thought deeply about making healthy food palatable. Dr. LaPuma is the author of *ChefMD's Big Book of Culinary Medicine: A Food Lover's Road Map to Losing Weight, Preventing Disease, and Getting Really Healthy*.[10] Given the data on the Mediterranean diet, I asked him how he would go about implementing this information. He said, "The Mediterranean diet [available here in Santa Barbara, where I am fortunate to practice] is the one eating pattern that appears to lower the risk for Alzheimer's dramatically, especially when compared with the Standard American diet. And the more Mediterranean you eat, the lower your risk, based on a study of 2,200 New Yorkers over four years. In fact, in another study, those with Alzheimer's who ate the most Mediterranean-type food lived up to four years longer than those who ate the least Mediterranean. What counts as Mediterranean?"

These are the three key points offered by Dr. LaPuma:

1. Vegetables, whole grains, fruits, nuts, olive oil, and fish are in the middle of the plate, daily.
2. Wine is a regular part of evening meals.
3. Red meat, poultry, rich dairy products, and highly processed cookies, candies, cakes, and sweets are rare: once weekly to once monthly.

It is unlikely that the Mediterranean diet will be the only diet that can reduce the risk for Alzheimer's disease. The overlap of cardiovascular risk factors and Alzheimer's risk factors suggests that other diets—perhaps those rich in fruits and vegetables—will also reduce the risk of Alzheimer's disease. For example, the rural Korean diet with its high proportion of vegetables may have similar effects.

Leafy greens are also a key ingredient for health. The vegetables that make the most difference are dark and green: chard, kale, arugula, and even spinach. The chemistry behind the health value of dark green vegetables is unknown, but current thinking is laying its bets on antioxidants in the greens. We do know that a common modification of proteins, called oxidation, can damage cells and becomes more frequent with aging. Oxidation is a chemical reaction that once begun can lead to a chain reaction that damages cells. Antioxidants block this chain reaction and prevent cell damage. Oxidation of certain proteins in the brain that reside in cell membranes may play a major part in how Alzheimer's disease develops. However, the chemical variety of the antioxidants is vast, and zeroing in on those that are most effective would be a worthy goal. Single vitamins, such as vitamins E, B-12, B-6, and folate, taken as pills do not appear sufficient to do the job, based on randomized trials.

An antioxidant in green tea appears to have beneficial effects on reducing the progression of Alzheimer's disease. A study of one thousand elderly Japanese people found that those who drank two small cups of green tea daily had half the cognitive impairment of those who drank three cups per week. Leafy green vegetables, which are a rich source of many antioxidants, are potentially more effective in preventing Alzheimer's disease. The strongest link between oxidation and a disease state is with cardiovascular disease. The overwhelming amount of data that tie Alzheimer's risk to the same factors that lead to cardiovascular disease forces the conclusion that antioxidants are worthy of study in Alzheimer's disease.

Fish is an important facet of the diet, and many people who eat fish (not counting fish sticks) have better memory protection than people who don't. Most researchers believe that the omega-3 fatty acids found in fish form the basis of the protection. Once again the origin of the association was the protective link to cardiovascular disease. In the 1970s researchers found that Greenland Eskimos consumed large amounts of fat from seafood, but displayed virtually no cardiovascular disease. The high level of omega-3 fatty acids in the seafood reduced triglycerides, heart rate, blood pressure, and atherosclerosis. Of the three common omega-3 fatty acids, DHA (docosahexaenoic acid) seems to be the most important in the brain. The best sources of DHA are salmon, mackerel, herring, anchovy, sardines, and trout. (Fish don't make DHA themselves. They get their omega-3 from the algae they eat, and there are now supplements of DHA made from algae available for those who don't like fish, or don't get enough of it.)

Beyond these all-too-brief nutritional pearls is a wealth of knowledge from those who are actually in the kitchen and know how to prepare food that is not only healthy but also tasty. Our point is that diet can reduce the likelihood of getting Alzheimer's disease. For many, that statement is not news. But how many of us accept the idea that every day we are making decisions about what we ingest that will affect our risk of getting Alzheimer's disease? As the days add up, the risks we incur become cumulative. Adhering to the best practices in terms of diet—even given our limited current knowledge—could affect many of the undesirable outcomes that lie in wait, particularly the loss of our ability to care for ourselves as cognitive impairment sets in. The right food choices now are much more effective in staving off Alzheimer's disease than any medication later on.

Often those preaching about healthy eating are a voice in the desert ridiculed by the voice in the dessert. The biggest challenge to healthy eating is the daily temptation of unhealthy food all around us. When you are hungry, the healthy choice on the menu is swamped by reams of unhealthy choices. A diet means steeling oneself to TV advertisements with sugary breakfasts and smiling children who never appear overweight, to magazine ads that have brought food photography to an art of psychological rendering more precise than that of the Dutch masters, and to fast-food outlets that are the only food option along most highways and in less affluent neighborhoods.

Parents may do their best to keep their children away from candy, but they are undermined by vending machines in the schools and, of course, by Halloween. Most doctors are neither trained in, nor particularly interested in, nutrition. From pesticides in agriculture to additives in the factory, the food industry is fundamentally a chemical industry—much like the paint industry. The chemical experimentation among food scientists is rarely related to health; their research for food chains, restaurants, and processed food manufacturers concerns food preservation, taste, and marketing.

What you choose to eat is a matter of habit built up over a lifetime. Habits, whether good or bad, are self-sustaining. Those who give up sweets or meats often lose their taste for them after a while and their temptation recedes. Important for Alzheimer's disease prevention, we need to think about the pathways to brain degeneration. The future is easy to disregard and hard to predict. But to believe blithely that you won't get the disease is unrealistic and to believe that your decisions today don't affect your chances is to fly in the face of overwhelming data. Alzheimer's disease is a disease of cumulative insults to the brain, and the best medicine we know for the disease is adopting prevention habits long before reaching the age of risk.

COGNITIVE CHALLENGES

The notion that exercising and challenging the brain will keep it functioning well is increasingly catching on. As a result, we are seeing a profusion of books with the mathematics puzzle Sudoku; and crossword puzzles may be one of the last reasons people hold on to their newspaper subscriptions. What is missing from this simplistic formula for cognitive health is a critical ingredient: the brain requires new challenges to maximize its activation. For example, as one becomes more expert at a video game, the amount of energy the brain uses to play the game decreases, as we described earlier with the game Tetris. In other words, with more skills the brain can accomplish the same goal with less energy. We have many examples of this phenomenon in everyday life. For example, first learning to drive a car requires total attention—likely using a lot of brain activity. Once we have been driving for a few years, the effort becomes so routine that we seek other distractions, such as the radio, conversation with a passenger, or talking on cell phone, as relief from the tedium. Likewise, those doing crossword puzzles for many years find that the challenge diminishes. For the brain, it is preferable to search for new challenges. "Using the brain" means engaging in challenges that activate or stimulate large regions of neurons in the brain.[11]

To place artificial challenges before us, several companies have designed computer programs that present increasingly difficult problems in memory and strategy. The user advances from level to level so that maximal brain activation is sustained. The list of these programs is extensive, targeting different ages and emphasizing different sensory systems, such as vision or hearing.

All these programs are objectively reviewed on the Web site Sharp-Brains. Some of earliest available games were Cognifit, Nintendo Brain Age, Brainware Safari, Posit Science, Cogmed, Fast ForWord, Happy Neuron, FitBrains, MyBrainTrainer, and Supermemo. Video games that activate those brain regions vulnerable to attack by Alzheimer's disease are the games we would want to play, and most of these games are likely to activate regions of the brain, such as the hippocampus, that are vulnerable to Alzheimer's disease. Some manufacturers claim their game activates areas related to strategic-planning ability in the frontal part of the brain, another region attacked in Alzheimer's disease.

Certainly, different video games have different brain activation patterns.[12] For example, in a comparison of Othello, Tetris, and Space Invader, functional magnetic resonance imaging (fMRI) in ten right-handed healthy participants showed increased activity in the prefrontal cortex, the premotor cortex, the parietal cortex, and the visual association cortex. However, Othello and Tetris, which require logical thinking, activated broader areas of the prefrontal cortex, and Space Invader and Tetris, which require real-time reaction, activated broader areas of the premotor and parietal cortexes.

What games can do fits well with the problem of mild cognitive impairment. First, read this description of some popular games for a young audience from a *New Yorker* article by Tom Bissell:

Super Mario requires an ability to recognize patterns, considerable hand-eye coordination, and quick reflexes. Gears requires the ability to think tactically and make subtle judgments based on scant information, a constant awareness of multiple variables (ammunition stores, enemy weaknesses) as they change throughout the game, and the spatial sensitivity to control one's movement through a space in which the "right" direction is not always apparent. . . . Often, there is no single way to accomplish a given task; improvisation is rewarded.[13]

Contrast this statement with a wonderful description of mild cognitive impairment by John Updike, also in the *New Yorker*:

[O]ld age he was discovering arrived in increments of uncertainty. Street signs, rearview mirrors, and one's own ability to improvise could no longer be trusted. He asked direction three times.[14]

If we accept that video games provide a cognitive boost, can stimulating activities prevent Alzheimer's disease or slow its course? To answer this question, the field needed to advance from studies that looked back at subjects and suggested that participation in cognitively stimulating activities in midlife might reduce the risk of Alzheimer's disease later on. What was needed were studies that follow a group of participants over many years, group them according to midlife cognitive activity and follow them to see if they eventually develop Alzheimer's disease. One of the most widely cited studies was done by investigators at the Rush-Presbyterian-St. Luke's Medical Center in Chicago.[15] They recruited older Catholic nuns, priests, and brothers from about forty groups across the United States. Eligibility for the study was age sixty-five years or older, absence of a clinical diagnosis of dementia, consent to annual clinical evaluations, and a willingness by participants to donate their brains for autopsy at the time of death. Of 1,003 people interested in the study, many were excluded by the eligibility criteria and ultimately 740 persons participated. They were examined annually for up to seven years, with the average participant being examined for 4.5 years. The generosity of the participants from various religious orders certainly contributed to our knowledge about Alzheimer's disease.

Participants were rated according to the amount of time they typically spent in seven common activities that involve information processing as a central component: viewing television; listening to radio; reading newspapers; reading magazines; reading books; playing games, such as cards or checkers, or doing crosswords or other puzzles; and going to museums. The list of what the investigators consider cognitive activity is a bit surprising, and even if we include television as a cognitive activity, we do not know from the study whether the viewer comprehended what he or she saw on the screen. Perhaps a better way to classify cognitive activity is whether it requires active responses to a variety of situations, like playing chess as opposed to reading a book. Nevertheless, the study was able to draw some interesting conclusions.

During the follow-up period, 111 developed a clinical condition diagnosed as Alzheimer's disease. Of this group, 51 have died, and brain autopsy results at the time of the study were available for 31 participants. Of these, 26, or 84 percent, were definitively diagnosed with Alzheimer's disease. On average, those participants who reported frequent cognitive activity when they entered the study were 47 percent less likely to develop Alzheimer's disease than those with infrequent activity. The investigators concluded that frequent cognitive activity in old age is associated with reduced risk of getting Alzheimer's disease.

The uniformity of the study population—clergy—is a strength because it tends to control for other variables that may affect more diverse populations, but it is also a weakness because we do not know whether the results apply to other population groups. So the same investigators published a second study in the same year of a biracial community in Chicago—and they came to the same conclusion.

Studies of this type quickly segue toward the question of whether the protection associated with cognitive exercise is possible at any stage of life. Lifelong engagement in cognitive challenges, beginning with high educational achievement, can unequivocally diminish the risk of Alzheimer's disease. Among the Chicago Catholic clergy, these same achievers may just be the ones who engage in more cognitive activity, and a lifetime of exercising the brain becomes its endowment in protecting one from Alzheimer's disease. The best-known study that supported brain endowment either from birth or during our early development as the basis for decreased risk for Alzheimer's disease once again tapped the religious community. In a series of fascinating publications, David Snowden, a professor in the Department of Neurology and the Sanders-Brown Center on Aging at the University of Kentucky Medical Center, followed older nuns from the School Sisters of Notre Dame throughout the United States. His work was funded by the National Institutes of Health beginning in 1990.[16]

One study Snowden conducted that did not rely on postmortem brain tissue was the review of autobiographical essays written by the nuns for their order when they were in their twenties at the time they took their vows. Sister Nicolette's autobiography, written when she was twenty, was packed full of thoughts. Here is an example from her essay: "After I finished the eighth grade in 1921 I desired to become an aspirant at Mankato but I myself did not have the courage to ask the permission of my parents so Sister Agreda did it in my stead and they readily gave their consent." Dr. Snowden measures sentences by their "idea density," and this one scores high. In contrast, another Mankato nun wrote in her essay, "After I left school, I worked in the post-office." Remarkably, the essays written by these nuns in their twenties were predictive of who would get Alzheimer's disease and who would escape. Those with the greatest idea density were more likely to escape the disease than those who expressed a paucity of ideas.

It is important to emphasize that the association with idea density in an essay at around age twenty and getting Alzheimer's disease more than five decades later is simply a statistical association. Anyone can get the disease. But because the odds favor those with essays rich in ideas and with more complex sentences, we can go to the next step and begin to think about the meaning of these findings—why would idea density at age twenty predict the likelihood of getting Alzheimer's disease?

The nun study and others that describe education as protective against getting Alzheimer's disease are interpreted by some to support the "brain reserve" hypothesis. According to this hypothesis, the nuns in both study groups get plaques and tangles at the same rate, but those who begin with a richer intellectual base are insulated to some extent from the clinical symptoms of the disease. In other words, the same number of plaques and tangles has less of an impact on an educated person than on a relatively uneducated person because the educated person has developed brain circuitry able to buffer him from a partial loss of function. The charge of a good scientist is not to become enamored with one's own hypothesis, but to search for inconsistencies and other explanations. In this case, perhaps education itself is not protective, but instead protection is due to higher socioeconomic status and education is simply a by-product of being wealthier. This possibility turned out not to be true. A study of a group of people in 1987 living in central Sweden, called the Kungsholmen Project, failed to find an association with socioeconomic status and concluded that one's socioeconomic status did not contribute to the increased likelihood of getting Alzheimer's disease among those with low levels of education.

An alternative idea is that using the brain has a more direct effect on the production of plaques and tangles. We know that brain stimulation increases the local blood flow to the region of the brain being stimulated. Along with the blood flow come those essential "brain goodies"—oxygen and glucose. Perhaps this enhanced metabolic support for the brain can stave off the Alzheimer plaques and tangles. The different tendencies toward Alzheimer's disease among the nuns seem inextricably linked to the aging process itself and individual differences in how we age. Dr. Snowden has pointed out that the nuns tend to live longer than other women, and in many convents there are a disproportionately high number of centenarians, often free of dementia. Although Snowden's findings about brain reserve are provocative, the underlying reasons for a long life among nuns are probably multifactorial, including what would lead one to the nunnery in the first place and their lifestyle within a strongly supportive community. In this setting the cumulative effects that lead to Alzheimer's disease appear to be reduced.

Cognitive interventions and education come in so many varieties that knowing what works and what does not work becomes imperative. The answer is simple—if the cognitive activity involves challenges, particularly new challenges, it can be effective. Music, yoga, learning a second language, travel—all can benefit the aging brain. Perhaps the best summary of what can work fits under the rather old-fashioned notion of adult education. All the video games, all the sudokus and crossword puzzles, are really just a poor substitute for the intellectual excitement of a learning environment. The gems of learning environments are our universities, where all the components for stimulating the brain—physical, mental, and social—are present in one place. Environments that value learning, such as universities, need to be more open and available to elders. Recently I was asked about implementing a lecture series in an assisted living community—and, of course, many such communities are already doing this. One member of the community told me he longed to hear a lecture on astronomy. How refreshing to find this thirst for knowledge among people who might otherwise simply drift into their sunset years with resignation and curiosity long since extinguished.

Our intellectual interests are even more diverse than the many types of diet or exercise programs available. After a career devoted to a demanding job, after raising a family, we may be drawn into the winding-down funnel of age. Without preparation it can be difficult to launch a new pursuit—just as at a younger age many temptations steal our time from practicing a musical instrument, from organizing in the community, from meeting the new people that lead to new activities. Just as we plan financially for retirement, we need to plan intellectually for retirement. For many, systematizing this planning in a center uniquely geared to thinking about the optimal next stage of life would be enormously beneficial. Without planning, we will be drawn into the lure of what the commercial interests would like us to do in our retirement years, like watching a steel roulette ball spin amid blinking lights in the casino. (Is it any accident that the suicide rate among elders is the highest in Las Vegas?)

FRIENDS

A growing body of data has found that a rich social network is a strong part of successful aging and likely to protect against Alzheimer's disease. Let's take a look at the Kungsholmen Project in Stockholm.[17] Beginning in 1987, all people age seventy-five or greater living in the district were asked to participate. Of 1,810 eligible participants, 1,473 had no evidence of dementia in clinical exams. This group was followed for the incidence of dementia. Participants were also classified according to activity categories: Mental activity included reading books/newspapers, writing, studying, working crossword puzzles, painting, or drawing. Physical activity included swimming, walking, or gymnastics. Social activity consisted of attending the theater, concerts, or art exhibitions; traveling; playing cards or games; or participating in social groups with other retirees. Productive activity was considered gardening, housekeeping, cooking, working for pay after retirement, doing volunteer work, sewing, knitting, crocheting, or weaving. Recreational activity included watching television or listening to the radio. The frequency of participation in activity was recorded as daily, weekly, monthly, or annually. The result: dementia incidence decreased with increasing frequency of participation in mental, physical, and social activities.

Many of the activities in these categories are social activities. To isolate the positive effects of social factors, another measure was developed. A person's social network was given a value based on marital status, the various people who lived together in the subject's home, parenthood, and close social ties that defined the structure of social connections. For each of these social connections, the examiners also gave a score for perceived adequacy, or how satisfying the subject found each component of his or her social network. Participants were classified in the two extremes: as having an extensive social network or as having a poor social network. An extensive social network consisted of being married or living with someone, having children and having daily to weekly satisfying contacts with them, and having relatives or friends and having daily to weekly satisfying contacts with them. A poor social network meant being single and living alone with no children and no close social ties. While a strong social network is of major importance, the three categories of activities all had beneficial effects independently of the strength of the social network as a whole. Taken together, this study and others suggest that a stimulating life, which includes participating in creative, educational, or interactive activities, may reduce the likelihood of developing dementia.

A more direct study of social engagement and cognitive decline was conducted by Lisa Berkman at the Harvard School of Public Health.[18] She studied a group from a site in New Haven, Connecticut, where the Established Populations for Epidemiologic Studies of the Elderly project is based. The sample population consists of 2,812 noninstitutionalized people sixty-five years of age or older who were living in New Haven in 1982. They were drawn from three types of housing situations: public housing for the elderly, private housing for the elderly, and community housing.

The study used indicators of social engagement: presence of a spouse; monthly visual contact with at least three relatives or close friends; yearly nonvisual contact—for example, telephone—with at least ten relatives or close friends; attendance at religious services at least once per month or membership in other groups; or regular participation in recreational social activities. The scores factored in the number of social ties each person in the study had. The emotional support that participants felt they could get from their social network was assessed by this question, "Can you count on anyone to provide you with emotional support—that is, talking over problems or helping make a difficult decision?"

The results were clear. Social disengagement was linked to the probability of cognitive decline when people were checked later. Those who were viewed as the least socially engaged were twice as likely to develop dementia as those participants in the study who were viewed as the most engaged. The social tie method of predicting cognitive decline also predicted higher death rates.

One of the closest social relationships is marriage. A report from the 2008 International Conference on Alzheimer's Disease in Chicago suggested that those who are unmarried or not living with a partner in midlife could have an increased risk of developing Alzheimer's disease. The study examined 1,449 individuals from the Finnish Cardiovascular Risk Factors, Aging, and Dementia Study in midlife conducted in the mid-1970s and then again in 1998, an average of twenty-one years later. When reexamined, 139 people were diagnosed with some form of cognitive impairment—82 with mild cognitive impairment and 48 with Alzheimer's disease.[19] Those who were living with a partner in midlife were significantly less likely to show cognitive impairment compared to those who were single, separated, divorced, or widowed. Those in the study who were married or lived with a significant other in midlife had a 50 percent lower risk of having dementia in late life compared to those who lived alone, even after adjustments for the usual confounding factors, including education, cholesterol, blood pressure, occupation, physical activity, smoking habits, depression, whether or not a participant has a gene linked to Alzheimer's disease known as APOE, age at follow-up, and gender.

A more detailed look at the group that was living alone showed that lifelong singles doubled their risk for Alzheimer's or mild cognitive impairment, those who stayed divorced from midlife onward tripled their risk, and those who were widowed before midlife and stayed widowed had a sixfold increased risk compared to those who were married at midlife and remained married in late life. These data provide strong support for the value of social relationships for lifelong brain health and point to one type of relationship—two people living together—as the highly effective means of reaping the benefits. The reasons for the beneficial effects are likely to be many—reduced stress by having someone else nearby, intellectual stimulation, and support of our basic social needs.

Certainly, a long marriage with many shared experiences is also an excellent memory aid. But as a couple in a long marriage move into retirement, the relationship may change and new stressors arise. I've heard many spouses lament, "I married him for life, not for lunch." On the other hand, little is more isolating and lonely than the death of a spouse. Coupled with the difficulty of meeting people in middle age and beyond, social isolation becomes increasingly likely. The barriers are high for those reentering the social scene after a divorce or the death of a spouse because just about everything in the dating game seems to trample upon long-established comforts. Enhancing the possibilities for social interactions might actually have an impact on Alzheimer's disease. A middle-aged person would certainly not turn to a physician for advice on dating, and yet satisfactory relationships are as important for good health as Pap smears and colonoscopies. In any case, the overburdened physician is not the answer. Instead, we need centers that encompass all the issues related to cognition, including social relationships. Just like trying to get medical advice from a Web site, going it alone on an online dating site, such as PlentyOfFish.com or PerfectMatch.com, can feel very impersonal. People just need a little bit of help in bringing together all the ingredients for good health, including structured settings that actively encourage new social relationships.

A bit of sage guidance can go a long way toward remedying a sense of isolation. A good first step is a counselor who can direct individuals to groups with shared interests from athletics to dancing to dining to community service. The list is very long. Second, we need to realize the vast diversity of relationships in which humans engage. What was important in dating and then in a relationship in your twenties may be less so now. What seems to be most important for mature daters is striking a balance between personal freedom and shared experience. No doubt this balance is important, but satisfaction can arrive in unexpected ways. I recall a couple in their early eighties who, a few years earlier, had met and married after both had been widowed for some time. He was blind and had trouble walking. Shortly after they were married, she developed Alzheimer's disease. He said to me, "Of course, I'll care for her. I'm old and blind. What else can I do?"

Social life is a highly nuanced matter that is practiced in vastly different ways—all with potentially equal satisfaction. Prescribing a specific type and level of social life for anyone based on a broad range of information would be a big mistake. Some people are quite satisfied with a very close relationship with one person. Others enjoy numerous acquaintances. At the extremes are isolated backwoods types or inspired loners who are neurologically tuned for isolation. Even more extreme are those on the high end of the autism spectrum, like Temple Grandin, the designer of livestock-handling facilities, who are not highly engaged with other humans but may experience something comparable to social engagement by interacting with animals. On the other hand, the loneliness that is so much a part of old age could be somewhat mitigated by developing community-based programs that promote social exchange and interaction.

CHRONIC STRESS—AN INNER TIME BOMB

Three lifestyle components—social, mental, and physical—appear to benefit a person's cognition and protect against dementia. These components also reduce stress. Chronic stress is very likely to contribute to cognitive decline, perhaps more so than any of the other factors we have discussed. The supportive data for this association is extensive, and we will discuss it here. The idea of emotional stress was formulated near the end of the 1940s by a Czech biochemist, Hans Selye, who adopted the term from metallurgy, as in the fine stress fractures found in airplane fuselages or wings after years of flying.[20] Unlike the lifestyle issues related to exercise and cognitive challenges, we have identified some of the key molecules that are biochemically involved.

The stress response involves an outpouring of steroid hormones called glucocorticoids as well as adrenalin. The stress reaction we feel sometimes is marvelously adaptive when we are faced with an acute threat like someone breaking into our home. Our muscles become stronger, as in those fabled cases of the parent who lifts an automobile to free a trapped child. Our blood pressure soars and our heart pounds. Even our thinking becomes clearer and the experience is burned into our memory. And everything that is unnecessary gets shut off—digestion, reproduction, fatigue—all in order to respond to the source of the stress. But when the threat, whether real or perceived, goes on and on, the same stress response becomes dangerous to our well-being. What was intended for an emergency is now turned on full time, and the negative consequences are huge.

If we are worrying about money or a failing marriage or an ill child or a problem at work, the glucocorticoids are flowing and eventually the body fails. Prolonged periods of stress can increase our risk of adult-onset diabetes, permanent high blood pressure, heart disease, infection, erectile dysfunction, menstrual cycle disruption, and gastrointestinal disorders. In the brain, those very neurons that become charged in an acute life-threatening encounter can wither and die from chronic stimulation. Many of those memory neurons reside in a brain structure called the hippocampus, the memory area of the brain that is one of the chief target regions of Alzheimer's disease. A definitive connection between Alzheimer's disease and the stress response does not exist, but the hypothesis is out there and needs to be taken seriously.

While the connection between stress and Alzheimer's disease remains tentative, animal experiments have strengthened the link. Frank LaFerla, a professor of neurobiology and behavior at the University of California at Irvine, genetically engineered a mouse to develop the plaques and tangles of Alzheimer's disease. Mice of this type are called transgenic, and the LaFerla mouse carries three human genes involved in Alzheimer's disease. The researchers injected four-month-old transgenic mice with levels of the glucocorticoid dexamethasone similar to the level of the hormone seen in humans under stress. After a treatment of just seven days, the levels of the protein in the senile plaque called beta-amyloid and the level of the protein in the neurofibrillary tangle called tau increased substantially. The connection to stress hormones implies that stress management should be part of an Alzheimer's treatment program, and patients should avoid glucocorticoids if possible.

Insights concerning stress have also come from years of fieldwork by Robert Sapolsky of Stanford University on African baboons in Kenya.[21] He makes the point that the success of some species in accumulating sufficient resources to relieve the need for constantly being in a survival mode has opened longer periods of time to develop a social consciousness. Sapolsky points out, "If you live in a baboon troop in the Serengeti, you only have to work three hours a day for your calories, and predators don't mess with you much. What that means is you've got nine hours of free time every day to devote to generating psychological stress toward other animals in your troop. So the baboon is a wonderful model for living well enough and long enough to pay the price for all the social-stressor nonsense that they create for each other. They're just like us: They're not getting done in by predators and famines, they're getting done in by each other."[22]

Sapolsky goes on to note that low-ranking baboons are highly susceptible to stress, as are Type A baboons. "Type A baboons are the ones who see stressors that other animals don't," according to Sapolsky. "For example, having your worst rival taking a nap 100 yards away gets you agitated." Then Sapolsky delivers the deep insight: "Up until 15 years ago, the most striking thing we found was that, if you're a baboon, you don't want to be low ranking, because your health is going to be lousy," he explains. "But what has become far clearer, and probably took a decade's worth of data, is the recognition that protection from stress-related disease is most powerfully grounded in social connectedness, and that's far more important than rank."[23]

Sapolsky pins many of our societal ills on stress. Ironically, although our living conditions are more crowded than at any time in our evolutionary history, we suffer from more isolation. Sapolsky points out, "Two of the healthiest states are Vermont and Utah, while two of the unhealthiest are Nevada and New Hampshire. Vermont is a much more left-leaning state in terms of its social support systems, while its neighbor New Hampshire prides itself on no income tax and go it alone. In Utah, the Mormon church provides extended social support. You can't ask for more than that. And next door is Nevada, where people are keeling over dead from all of their excesses." Getting along with those around us is part of a healthy lifestyle. As Sapolsky has quipped, "What's the punch line here? Physiologically, it doesn't come cheap being a bastard twenty-four hours a day."[24]

Chronic stress is a significant risk factor for ill health, including impairment of brain function. Nearly all formulas for stress reduction involve lifestyle modifications. While we do not have good data on the success rate of stress-reduction regimens, the data that do exist suggest that this approach can have a significant impact on preventing cognitive decline late in life. A surprising variety of inroads to stress reduction exists—the problem is to implement these lifestyle changes consistently. Although it may seem simplistic, the facts are unmistakable: the principle approaches to stress reduction are exercise, restful sleep, enjoyment of friends and relationships, and entry into relaxing mental states.

A fundamental principle of biology is homeostasis—the internal balance of body and mind. The recognition of this principle is attributed to a towering nineteenth-century French scientist, Claude Bernard, who wrote, "*La fixité du milieu intérieur est la condition d'une vie libre et indépendante*" ("The constancy of the internal environment is the condition for a free and independent life").[25] With chronic stress and the release of hormones related to the fight-or-flight response, the body resets its baseline hormonal levels to that of a stressed state.

An intense workout sets up a different pattern. Exercise is also a stressor that increases blood pressure, heart rate, and adrenalin, but after a bout of exercise the body restores itself to a lower baseline state and prepares for future surges of stress. Exercise also increases the core temperature of the body, which induces a response to the release of heat by dilating blood vessels, thereby warming the whole body. Consequently, blood pressure is reduced and tissues throughout the body receive more oxygen. Exercise also can alleviate depression, which dulls cognition.

Some form of sleep is a universal need for any organism with a brain, and even short periods of sleep deprivation can be stressful. Chronic inadequate sleep increases the risk of depression, diabetes, obesity, and cardiovascular disease, and impairs cognitive function. Ultimately, long-term sleep deprivation leads to a collapse of the immune system and death by infectious disease. A single night of poor sleep increases the tendency of the body to produce the toxic substances that fight-off infection but can also damage the body when produced in excess. This reaction to stress is called an inflammatory response, and chronic inflammation is tied to many aspects of aging and nearly all the chronic diseases associated with aging. Individuals differ in their sleep requirements, even within the same family. Most people require six to eight hours per night; however, a very small group of people who require less sleep have a mutation in a sleep-control gene. This finding has led some researchers to speculate that the best answer to the question of how much sleep we need will differ from person to person and depend on small changes in our genes. Nevertheless, for most of us, if we get fewer than five and a half hours of sleep, our thinking suffers and our inflammatory markers and health risks rise.

But even these generalities can be misleading because one must also consider the quality of the sleep: eight hours of fitful sleep can be worse than five hours of deep, restorative sleep. Time in bed is less important than time spent in restorative sleep. Dream sleep is restorative as a time when we consolidate memories and enhance creativity, learning, problem solving, and emotional balance. During dreaming the brain has got its power level set on high—it is devoting lots of energy toward the restorative functions. Deep sleep is when the brain slows down and is a time for physical rather than psychic repair. During deep sleep the body secretes growth hormone to assist in its own repair.

In our effort to get more sleep, we are once again up against the power of social forces. Just as our attempts to eat right are undermined by advertisements for junk food, sleeping is widely viewed as only for slackers. Much of our effort directed toward a healthy lifestyle will require a broad social buy-in to overcome the barrage of phony lifestyles we see presented to us by the commercial media.

As we have noted, a rich social network is perhaps the number one predictor of successful aging. Once again social isolation takes its toll on the immune system. Of course, social isolation is a relative matter and often quite subjective—one close friend can be preferable to a wide circle of acquaintances. When social isolation is used as a predictor for successful aging, the best measurement is one's own perception of social isolation and feelings of loneliness. The effects of feeling lonely are profound—they even affect our genes.[26] In a group of people who reported feeling very lonely, two hundred nine genes were altered, either more turned on or more turned off, than in the control population. Among the altered genes were several that control the immune system. A special category of social relationship is love between two people. Although the nature of these special relationships varies greatly, they are beneficial for the brain. A deep, intimate connection buffers one's response to stress. Supporting data include lower levels of adrenaline and cortisol, a hormone produced by the adrenal gland that is known as "the stress hormone," in married people. Married people generally live longer than single people, and the marriage effect is greater for men than for women. Conflict in a marriage more than cancels any positive effects and becomes a powerful stressor.

Purposefully seeking a relaxing mental state is a highly effective means of reducing stress. The techniques for mental relaxation are as diverse as those for child rearing. And, as in child rearing, most of them work, and they work even better if the relaxation technique fits with one's own interests and preferences. Yoga, meditation, deep breathing, or watching a sunset can all create a brain state conducive to cognitive health. During meditation heart rate, blood pressure, and stress hormones all drop, and baseline levels for all these risks drop with regular meditation. Mindfulness, or focusing on the present moment, is key to all the techniques. Of course, the present moment is forever evanescent, so remaining still in a river of time is challenging.

Equally challenging is avoiding what might be a called a worry loop or the inability to detach one's thoughts from a particular concern. Instead, the mind loops round and round on the same problem, like coming back again and again to scratch an itch. Techniques like chanting a mantra or taking regular, deep breaths are designed to break the loop and help participants remain focused.

THE HAPPINESS SOLUTION

We have learned that once one gets beyond a certain minimum level of poverty, more money is not terribly useful in relieving stress. Nor does money buy a great deal of happiness, the best stress reliever we know. Again, the exception is those in abject poverty, for whom a small amount can make a huge difference in happiness. For many, however, despite wealth, stress-related diseases remain common. More important, wealth does not appear to be the way to escape from these ailments. Perhaps to the detriment of our health, governments spend a large proportion of their efforts in building wealth when they could be more effective if they concentrated on building happiness. Of course, there is some overlap between the two, but having one's priorities in order would make a big difference.

Happiness is front and center in the words of the Declaration of Independence, which argues for "certain inalienable Rights, that among these are Life, Liberty and the Pursuit of Happiness, " as well as in the moral philosophy of Jeremy Bentham and other utilitarians, who argued that the purpose of politics should be to bring the greatest happiness to the greatest number of people. It also is the subject of a 2006 British survey, which reported that 81 percent of the population believed the government's primary objective should be the creation of happiness not wealth.[27]

Evaluating governments based on the happiness they create among their people has received considerable attention from economists. To do so we need an objective measurement of happiness, a gross national happiness (GNH) that has comparable precision to the gross national income (GNI). As early as the 1970s, the Kingdom of Bhutan proclaimed that it wanted to maximize gross national happiness rather than gross national income. Happiness researchers (not necessarily the same as happy researchers) have devised measuring tools to quantify subjective well-being. These include global evaluations of individual life satisfaction; the Experience Sampling Method, which collects information on individuals' actual experience in real time in their natural environments; the Day Reconstruction Method, which asks people to reflect on how satisfied they felt at various times during the day; the U ("unpleasant")-Index, defined as the fraction of time per day that an individual spends in an unpleasant state; and brain imaging, to scan individuals' brain activities for correlates of positive and negative affect.

Except for collecting global evaluations of individual life satisfaction, taking these measurements is time consuming and expensive. So much of the data rely on global evaluations of individual life satisfaction. This simple measuring method is considered reliable because it reveals that happy people smile more often during social interactions; are rated as happy by friends, spouses, and family members; express positive emotions more frequently; are more optimistic; are more sociable and extraverted; sleep better; and are also less likely to commit suicide. The measure also observes the Easterlin paradox: that while real per capita income has dramatically increased in many countries, happiness has remained constant.

Bruno S. Frey and Alois Stutzer incisively discuss the maximizing of aggregate happiness as an objective of public policy. They point out that a key tenet of happiness research is found in the many changes in life circumstances that have only a short-lived effect on reported subjective well-being because people adapt to the new situation.[28] Commonly cited examples of what has been called hedonic, or pleasure, adaptation are paraplegics. If asked before an accident that leaves a person paraplegic how he or she would feel after becoming paralyzed, people tend to report a degree of sadness that borders on being suicidal. "I would kill myself if I became totally paralyzed," is a common reaction to the thinking about this possibility. But, in fact, after a period of struggle, most paraplegics report themselves long term to be only a little less happy than before. Likewise lottery winners, after a short period of elation, report themselves to be not much happier than before. Another behavioral motivator that tends to remain constant is a person's aspirations. People quite rapidly adjust to increases in income so that, after about one year, two-thirds or more of the benefits of an increase in income wear off as people increase their income aspirations. This phenomenon is called the aspiration treadmill. These human traits make maximizing aggregate happiness difficult.[29]

Countries show great variation in self-reported happiness. While all these studies have to be interpreted cautiously, Denmark, with its democracy, social equality, and peaceful atmosphere, is ranked the happiest country, while the world's richest nation, the United States, is sixteenth, according to the US government-funded World Values Survey.[30] Also ranked highly are Colombia, Puerto Rico, Northern Ireland, Switzerland, Ireland, the Netherlands, Canada, and Sweden. None of these countries have expansive happiness programs, so what accounts for the differences? The stark economic differences between Haiti and the Dominican Republic are reflected in the happiness of their inhabitants. But once we control for economic differences, happiness differences are harder to explain. In Colombia dancing is much more common than in the United States. Almost any social gathering of any age group might have dancing, even in very limited space. Do they dance because they are happy or does the dancing make them happy? More generally, attributing the happiness differences to undefinables such as national character does not really explain the basis for the differences.

No doubt the implementation of a happiness program at the level of government is neither desirable nor practical. We really do not want a government to force changes of preference on its citizens. We don't want the government deciding what makes us happy and then forcing the "happiness pill" down our throats. From the government's perspective, happiness may not be the ultimate goal. The government may want to instill loyalty, responsibility, self-esteem, freedom, or personal development as much as happiness. A better place to aim the findings of happiness research is the healthcare community. In this setting, there is more opportunity to distinguish individual well-being from aggregate happiness. Individuals should be able to advance their own ideas of the good life, rather than maximizing the good of all.

Including knowledge about happiness research when reviewing the healthcare system is long overdue. First, chronic stress is harmful to our health. Second, the best stress reliever is happiness. That is easy enough to say, but it can be hard to achieve. Nevertheless, if we want to have an impact on Alzheimer's disease and we want to adopt lifestyles that can delay the onset of the disease, it would behoove us to know something about happiness. And the person to ask is Harvard professor Dan Gilbert. Professor Gilbert has a gift for walking directly into a nest of problems with the ease and grace of a magician whose logic brings clarity to human foibles. In his book *Stumbling on Happiness*, he puts forth a central idea—that people are very poor about predicting what will make them happy and as a result make some very bad decisions.[31] We get failing grades in predicting our own happiness because our ability to imagine future events is infested with inaccuracies and details that are added or removed. We tend not to take into account that fundamentally we just don't change that much, and therefore what looks to be transformative will likely turn out to be not so different from the past. In my own case, every time I see a sleek sailboat with its full sails gliding across a perfect seascape, I am drawn in and would readily accept an invitation to get on board. But I also know from personal experience that once on board with the sun beating down and the unchanging monotony of water and sky, boredom would set in. Even though I know full well that the outing would probably be tedious, it always remains attractive and I remain vulnerable to repeating the error again and again. Gilbert believes that we can get a better read on decisions that affect our future happiness by consulting others and not relying solely on our own often-misdirected instincts. If someone knows you well, then a timely reminder of what the imagined experience will actually be like is all you may need.

So if we are so poor at predicting what will make us happy, are there some general guidelines, is there some yardstick against which we can measure the rash decisions based on an illusory future? Probably for most people, the best predictors of happiness are human relationships and the amount of time that people spend with family and friends. Often people sacrifice social relationships for something that is far less likely to bring happiness. The culprit is often money, but also on the list are power and sex. But remember that the pitch here is not a moral one—important as that is—it is a selfish one. Usually, but not always, your happiness can be enhanced by friends and family more than other options that may be tempting. In general, measures of happiness include nonmaterial aspects of human well-being, such as the influence of social relations, autonomy, and self-determination. Dan Gilbert points out that experiences bring more happiness than material things. So the advice is, when you have a choice, choose vacations or movies over a new handbag or jewelry or a sports car. From experiences we get memories, and these are more permanent than objects. Too often we fall for the "diamonds are forever" myth. Without the relationship that the diamond signifies, the stone left behind can be a cruel reminder.

All the lifestyle factors we have discussed reduce one's risk for getting Alzheimer's disease. As years go by while one ignores these risk factors, cumulative damage to the brain mounts. Once that damage reaches a threshold, clinical symptoms of memory loss and personality change set in. At this point, interventions have little effect on the inexorable progression of the disease. One cannot start too early to begin to reduce risk and adopt protective measures. Diet and exercise are matters of habit and much easier to do once the habit is established. Keeping the mind active, gathering friends, and keeping stress at bay are all lifelong goals. The idea behind the neighborhood cognitive shop, as discussed in chapter 2, is to have a place that helps instill these brain health habits.

SOCIAL NETWORKS DRIVE ADHERENCE

Nearly all physicians agree that one of the biggest obstacles to better health is the difficulty of adhering to healthy practices. People know quite a bit about a healthy lifestyle, but finding the discipline to adhere to what they know is very difficult. Just taking a daily pill, like a medication for a seizure disorder or an antibiotic, is frequently ignored. Adherence becomes so much more of a problem when it requires major behavioral changes in diet or exercise patterns. What has become very clear is that behaviors, whether positive or negative, can be changed through social networks. The health sector needs to take better advantage of this behavioral approach for improving the health of the community.

The strength of social factors in health has vividly broken into the medical literature with the finding by Nicholas Christakis and James Fowler, who suggested that friends have an even more important effect on a person's risk of obesity than genes do. By reconstructing all the social links among friends, neighbors, spouses, and family members of participants in the Framingham Heart Study, a study of a large group of patients over three generations in Framingham, Massachusetts, by the National Heart, Lung, and Blood Institute and Boston University, the authors observed that when two persons perceived each other as friends, if one friend became obese during a set time interval, the other friend's chances of also becoming obese increased by 171 percent.[32] Pairs of adult siblings had a lower risk of passing along obesity—if one sibling became obese, the chance that the other would become obese increased by 40 percent. Thus, the influence of friends was greater than that of family.[33]

In the obesity social network, the risk that the friend of a friend of an obese person would be obese was about 20 percent higher in the observed network than in a random network. By the fourth degree of separation, the effect vanished. The same authors who did the obesity study again used the Framingham Heart Study to look for similar network effects on smoking. Within this densely interconnected network of

12,067 people who were assessed repeatedly from 1971 to 2003, Christakis and Fowler looked at person-to-person spread of smoking behavior and the extent to which groups of widely connected people quit together.

Just to get an idea of the enormous size of the study, the investigators assembled 53,228 family and social ties among 5,124 subjects. On average, each person had 10.4 ties to other members, not including ties to neighbors. Most often, these ties were spouses and siblings. Given the decades of time over which they could observe changes in the network, the authors found that some fascinating changes emerged. Not only did many people stop smoking (not surprising), but the remaining smokers tended to get pushed to the periphery of the network. To understand what that means, think of networks as organized around hubs. A hub is a person who has lots of connections to other people in the network, and hubs lie in the center of the network. Think about flight patterns and an airline hub. Those people with few connections lie at the periphery like a small, remote town with one flight in and one flight out. In this study, smokers became increasingly isolated. And the smokers formed their own clusters, with many fewer connections between smokers and nonsmokers than among the smokers themselves. To put actual numbers on these connections among smokers, the average risk of being directly connected to a smoker (one degree of separation) was 61 percent higher in the actual network than in a random network. The risk of being a smoker was 29 percent higher for contacts' contacts (at two degrees of separation) and 11 percent higher for contacts' contacts' contacts (at three degrees of separation). By the fourth degree of separation, the effect vanished, as in the obesity study. In general, the reach of the smoking clusters was three degrees. These data could not be explained by coincident clustering due to socioeconomic factors.

For the final point, picture clusters of smokers. They know each other, but there are very few connections between clusters of smokers. In other words, you know your smoker friends but not other smokers who have their own set of smoker friends. Over time, as the total number of smokers declines, those who stop smoking do not stop evenly from all the clusters. Instead, smoking declines by entire clusters—at some threshold a large number of people abruptly shift their behavior and stop smoking. Fashion works similarly in the way that a new style spreads. Friends influence each other, sometimes over two or three degrees of separation, in smoking cessation. Friendships could be mutual or unidirectional, in that you may consider someone your friend but that person does not consider you a friend. Mutual friendships had more influence on smoking cessation than unidirectional friendships. As behavior changes in a network, some people may have more influence than others, and they are called opinion leaders. Identifying opinion is important when attempting to change behavior.

As pointed out by Christakis and Fowler, the network or group phenomena might be exploited to spread many positive health behaviors. The power of the person-to-person spread of smoking cessation might be harnessed to reduce other harmful behaviors. In the case of Alzheimer's disease, we have identified some maladaptive behaviors that increase the risk of getting the disease. These include lack of exercise, poor diet, cognitive lethargy, and the presence of cardiovascular risk factors. How, then, can we go about applying social network principles to reduce the incidence of Alzheimer's disease? Step one is to begin long before anyone has the symptoms of Alzheimer's disease—the disease must be prevented before it gains a foothold.

Therefore, look to webs of social networks that surround all of us based on some shared activity—whether it is going to the same shopping center, belonging to the same church group, being alumni of the same college, or joining a special interest Web site. These are networks of middle-aged people—people at an age that might be considered the last stop before the die is cast and the cumulative effects of risk put one on a collision course with the disease.

In the case of the smoking cessation study, the shared activity was participation in a large medical study geographically centered in Framingham, Massachusetts. Many participants lived relatively near the study site. If our goal is to reduce the incidence of Alzheimer's disease using social networks, then one way to begin assembling the network will be to link people locally who are motivated to seek out preventive measures. Placing cognitive shops in communities is ideal for nucleating social networks—that is, identifying a set of early adopters whose friends and then their friends begin to grow a large and complex network of social interactions. Cognitive shops, described in chapter 2, house in one location all the services known to prevent or delay late-life cognitive decline. Because the risk of getting Alzheimer's disease is so high, practicing prevention is for everyone, long before they develop any symptoms, and the cognitive shop makes it possible to implement a prevention program in the community available to everyone.

Once a loosely knit, community-based interest group is formed around the problem of preserving cognition and grows from the networked connections of those who visit the local cognitive shop, we will need to create environments that can drive healthy behavior. Many people know what constitutes healthy behaviors, but they do not do it. The reasons for this are complex and involve motivation, discipline, and the influence of peers and the media. In the Framingham Heart Study network, smoking cessation was passively driven by the overall societal rejection of smoking. In an Alzheimer prevention network, the drivers will need to be more active mainly because the behavioral change is not the cessation of a habit, but the adoption of a new habit. In the case of diet, we need to substitute a healthier one for current eating habits. Creating an actively driven network would utilize the social networking features of Facebook, the Web site that creates virtual networks of friends, to build a health-oriented site. Facebook allows people, who are willing, to observe each other's efforts in adopting those lifestyles that reduce risk. The success of one's friends in the network is the behavioral driver.

Users enter what they've eaten, the time they've spent exercising, and the time they've spent doing cognitive fitness games. Users can see similar data on their friends. Aggregate data is assembled through the site and presented to the group. In other words, members of the site will be able to see the collective achievements of the group. The site will also offer goals to motivate the entire group toward optimal behaviors and avoid rebel network effects that drive the user group toward risky behaviors. Of course, the accuracy of entered data is always a question because sometimes people lie. As technology advances, however, an interface between a stationary bicycle or an elliptical in the gym and the site can provide documentation of the entered data, and already time spent on cognitive games can be tracked online. Cell phone scanners that read bar codes on food labels and compute calories and nutritional value could help with data entry.

Some networks might agree to be more revealing of personal data, such as blood pressure, weight (or more appropriately, a weight that is normalized for height), cholesterol level, and current medications. The accuracy of data can be enhanced by direct entry through an Internet-connected device that measures blood pressure or glucose or travels through a seamless link from a lab that measures lipid levels to the Internet site. In contrast to young Facebook users who are curious about each other's wardrobes, party invitations, and the biggest buzz item of all—relationship status—many elders are interested in each other's medical data. Often health-related topics completely dominate conversations among retirees. The motive for logging into a "Facebook for seniors" will be medical updates about each other, as well as personalized health tips from a recommender feed. For example, a high blood pressure reading might generate an alert or a steep drop in time spent exercising might generate an inquiry or new dietary information might appear as an RSS feed (Really Simple Syndication is a format to deliver frequently updated information to Web sites). Just as with lifestyle data, medical data will also be aggregated and made available to the group. In this way, the network will have some sense of how they are collectively doing on those medical measurements that predict lifelong cognitive health. With network data in hand, doctors will be able to target their interventions to virtual locales defined by social connections.

All entered information would be dated and would expire after a set time interval, with an update request sent to the user. Over time, the site will assess changes in all the parameters measured—it will track individual changes and group changes and notify the network as members' health risks diminish. In this way the online social network will bring group pressure on individuals to adhere to healthy behaviors, a team sense of accomplishment, and a highly informed user group with richer social links to others.

Because medical data is quite sensitive and may be more or less sensitive for some, the site will offer users the option either to allow or not allow others to view any particular parameter. For example, someone may not want the group to know her weight, but will allow her weight to be computed in the group statistics. She would enter her weight and simply click not to allow her weight to be seen by the group. Or someone may be willing to share his data with his immediate friends, but not with friends of friends, that is, higher degrees of separation. The site will thus allow a close-up look at those people we know best, and as one dials out to more distant relationships, the user will only see aggregate data. For example, among your own friends, you might find that everyone is quite trim and exercising every day, but among more distant groups—those you do not directly—the numbers may be less good. However, over time your group's success may ripple through the network and the numbers among more distant users will improve.

NOTES

1. "Lifestyle Factors Contribute to Raising and Lowering Risk of Alzheimer's Disease," *Medical News Today*, July 31, 2008, http://www.medicalnewstoday.com/articles/116698.php.

2. J. Weuve et al., "Physical Activity, including Walking, and Cognitive Function in Older Women," Nurses' Health Study, *Journal of the American Medical Association* 292, no. 12 (2004): 1454–61.

3. R. D. Abbott et al., "Walking and Dementia in Physically Capable Elderly Men," *Journal of the American Medical Association* 292, no. 12 (2004): 1447–53.

4. Y. Netz et al., "Physical Activity and Psychological Well-Being in Advanced Age: A Meta-Analysis of Intervention Studies," *Psychological Aging* 20, no. 2 (2005): 272–84.

5. E. B. Larson et al., "Exercise Is Associated with Reduced Risk for Incident Dementia among Persons 65 Years of Age and Older," *Annals of Internal Medicine* 144, no. 2 (2006): 73–81; L. J. Podewils et al., "Physical Activity, APOE Genotype, and Dementia Risk: Findings from the Cardiovascular Health Cognition Study," *American Journal of Epidemiology* 161(2005): 639–51.

6. N. T. Lautenschlager et al., "Effect of Physical Activity on Cognitive Function in Older Adults at Risk for Alzheimer Disease: A Randomized Trial," *Journal of the American Medical Association* 300, no. 9 (September 3, 2008): 1027–37. For guidelines on general physical activity, see US Department of Health and Human Services, "Healthy People 2010"; Centers for Disease Control and Prevention, "Prevalence of Physical Activity, including Lifestyle Activities among Adults—United States, 2000–2001," *Morbidity and Mortality Weekly Report* 52 (2003): 764–69. For more on exercise and brain regions, see A. C. Pereira et al., "An In Vivo Correlate of Exercise-Induced Neurogenesis in the Adult Dentate Gyrus," *Proceedings of the National Academy of Science* 104 (2007): 5638–43.

7. S. J. Colombge et al., "Aerobic Fitness Reduces Brain Tissue Loss in Aging Humans," *Journal of Gerontology: Medical Sciences* 58 (2003): 176–80. Also see S. Colombe and A. F. Kramer, "Fitness Effects on the Cognitive Function of Older Adults: A Meta-Analytic Study," *Psychological Science* 14 (2003): 125–30.

8. For more on the Mediterranean diet and Alzheimer's, see *Annals of Neurology* 59, no. 6 (June 2006): 912–21.

9. N. Scarmeas et al., "Physical Activity, Diet, and Risk of Alzheimer Disease," *Journal of the American Medical Association* 302, no. 6 (August 12, 2009): 627–37.

10. John LaPuma, *ChefMD's Big Book of Culinary Medicine: A Food Lover's Road Map to Losing Weight, Preventing Disease, and Getting Really Healthy* (New York: Crown, 2008).

11. R. S. Wilson et al., "Participation in Cognitively Stimulated Activities and Risk of Incident Alzheimer Disease," *Journal of the American Medical Association* 287 (2002): 742–48.

12. K. Saito and M. Saito, "Brain Activity Comparison of Different-Genre Video Game Players," *Innovative Computing, Information and Control*, Second International Conference (September 2007): 402.

13. Tom Bissell, "Games—The Grammar of Fun," *New Yorker*, November 3, 2008, p. 78.

14. John Updike, "Free," *New Yorker*, January 8, 2000.

15. More on the study can be found at http://www.rush.edu/rumc/page -1099611542043.html.

16. Mark Stibich, "Aging with Grace: The Nun Study," About.com; see also http://nihseniorhealth.gov/alzheimersdisease/faq/video/a4_transcript.html for more on Snowden's work.

17. The study can be found at http://www.kungsholmenproject.se/.

18. S. S. Bassuk et al., "Social Disengagement and Incident Cognitive Decline in Community-Dwelling Elderly Persons," *Annals of Internal Medicine* 131 (1999): 165–73.

19. Todd Neale, "Marriage May Protect Against Dementia," *MedPage Today*, July 30, 2008, http://www.medpagetoday.com/MeetingCoverage/ ICAD/10334.

20. Erin O'Donnell, "Does Thinking Make It So?" *Harvard Magazine*, January–February 2009.

21. "Robert Sapolsky Discusses Physiological Effects of Stress: We've Evolved to Be Smart Enough to Make Ourselves Sick," *Stanford Report*, March 7, 2007, http://news-service.stanford.edu/news/2007/march7/sapolskysr-0307 07.html.

22. Ibid.

23. Ibid.

24. Ibid.

25. J. Kryspin, "Homeostasis: From Claude Bernard to Quantum Physics," *Canadian Medical Association Journal*, July 17, 1977, http://www .pubmedcentral.nih.gov/articlerender.fcgi?artid=1879618.

26. H. X. Wang et al., "Friends and Alzheimer's," *American Journal of Epidemiology* 155, no. 12 (June 15, 2002): 1081–87.

27. M. Easton, "Britain's Happiness in Decline," July 21, 2006, http:// www.news.bbc.co.uk/1/hi/programmes/happiness_formula.

28. Bruno S. Frey and Alois Stutzer, "What Can Economists Learn from Happiness Research?" Center for Economic Studies and Ifo Institute for Economic Research, Swiss Federal Institute of Technology, Zurich, June 2002, CESifo Working Paper Series No. 503; Zurich IEER Working Paper No. 80.

29. Daniel Kahneman and Alan B. Kreuger, "Developments in the Measurement of Subjective Well-Being," *Journal of Economic Perspectives* 20, no. 1 (2006): 3–24; also see Working Paper No. 306, "Should National Happiness Be Maximized?" March 2007; Shane Frederick and George Loewenstein, "Hedonic Adaptation," in *Well-Being: The Foundation of Hedonic Psychology*, ed. Daniel Kahneman, Ed Diener, and Norbert Schwarz (New York: Russell Sage Foundation, 1999), pp. 302–329.

30. The World Values Survey can be found at http://www.worldvalues survey.org/.

31. Daniel Gilbert, *Stumbling on Happiness* (New York: Vintage, 2007).

32. Information about the Framingham Heart Study can be found at http://www.framinghamheartstudy.org/.

33. N. A. Christakis and J. H. Fowler, "Social Networks and Obesity: The Spread of Obesity in a Large Social Network Over 32 Years," *New England Journal of Medicine* 357 (2007): 370–79; N. A. Christakis and J. H. Fowler, "Smoking and Social Networks," *New England Journal of Medicine* 358, no. 21 (May 22, 2008): 2249–58.

10

CONCLUSIONS

Sometimes attaining the deepest familiarity with a question is our best substitute for actually having the answer.
—Brian Greene, professor of mathematics and physics, Columbia University

Just as the idea of hospice care revolutionized death and dying in America, the idea of bundling many aspects of Alzheimer's care under one roof in a cognitive shop could change the way we approach this dire disease—one that has no cure and leaves no survivors.

Certainly, the scope of the problem poses medical and economic risks for the country. These risks, and potential steps for a solution, were charted by the bipartisan Alzheimer Study Group in the spring of 2009. The report, issued by the Alzheimer Study Group cochaired by former congressman Newt Gingrich and former senator Bob Kerrey, minces few words. It likens the failure to address the impact of Alzheimer's to the failure to strengthen the levies of New Orleans against an overwhelming hurricane.

"Alzheimer's is having a large and quickly growing medical and economic impact on the country, no significant medical treatments exist to halt this trend, and our healthcare system is not delivering adequate care to many of those with Alzheimer's and their caregivers."[1] Among other recommendations, the study group called for an Alzheimer's czar to coordinate policy.

As the baby boomers reach the age when Alzheimer's can begin to take hold, the committee is right to sound an alarm. The fractious debate about healthcare reform, with the overarching questions about the role of private insurers versus the government, is broad by necessity, and cannot address the changes needed in a fragmented system of care for long-term diseases like Alzheimer's.

Physicians are boxed in by an insurance system that pays them a fee for every service rendered, yet does not pay for time spent with a patient's family outlining a plan for diet, fitness, and social services like respite care. Patients and families find themselves pasting together a complicated network of care on their own, getting referrals to community social service agencies, transportation services, adult daycare, overnight care, and support groups. Accompanying a partner or a spouse with Alzheimer's to appointment after appointment is hard on elders; the situation can be even more nightmarish for the spouse of a patient with early onset Alzheimer's. Although early onset is a much rarer form of Alzheimer's, it poses unique burdens: the patient's spouse may still be working outside the home and tending to school-age children.

In short, Alzheimer's disease has been wedged into a medical system that has no place for it. Patients and their families can easily get lost in a labyrinthine empire, built up over years as healthcare became more costly and more regimented, and as science struggled to move beyond outdated ideas.

The hospice movement involved recalibrating the care of patients at the end of their lives, putting their needs first. It meant viewing care as a whole, not just a sum of tests, procedures, tubes, and bedside monitors. It meant a new emphasis on pain relief and humanity, while providing families the opportunity for relief from round-the-clock care of a dying loved one. Before hospice, death of a loved one often took place in a stark hospital room, amid a tangle of beeping electronic gear and tubes delivering medicine that was no longer effective. Family members wedged in visits, and nurses and doctors often bustled in and out, administering procedures that did little to alter the overall prognosis. After hospice care became accepted in the mainstream of medicine, the individuality of patients and families was taken into consideration—their wishes, their fears, their emotions. Measures of comfort, often delivered by professionals who were not doctors, became important.

Community-based cognitive centers could usher in similar changes in Alzheimer's care—with an important difference. A cognitive center would not be a place to go to die, but a place to find support and information. Based in a patient's neighborhood, not in an imposing academic hospital in a big city, the cognitive shop would offer a sort of one-stop shopping for everything from Alzheimer's disease prevention to guided care for mild or moderate disease.

Think about the dentist's office as an analogy: dental offices are found all over, not just in hospitals, and provide a fairly complete menu of care without the need for expensive specialists. When necessary, a dentist refers a patient to an endodontist or another specialist, but she generally treats most conditions in the office—and dentists and other staff, like hygienists, deliver preventive care in the same setting.

The cognitive shop would provide support for physicians, too, by reducing the focus and the burden on a single doctor. A wide array of questions from families and patients could be answered by a social services worker or by a patient Navigator, who would guide them to existing points of information. Families would be shown how to find support groups or tap into computerized information right there at the center. Patients would not have to shuttle across town after diagnosis to an expensive specialist like a neurologist, and then make additional appointments for therapy, for example. Spouses could get a needed break so they could go to work or shop or visit friends—generally refreshing their own support network.

There is another parallel to the hospice movement in the low-tech solutions that could be housed in the cognitive shop. The staff could also provide low-tech tests for people who wondered if they were beginning to slide into dementia—a service that could help cut down on expensive tests like MRI scans for people complaining of memory loss. A nurse or a physician's assistant could take histories and information's from patients, administer memory tests, take blood pressure and other samples if needed, and provide information about social services. Medical doctors could be brought in only when needed, shifting some of the burden from the overworked physician—an important shift given the shortage of primary-care doctors.

What will the cognitive shop look like? Consider this hypothetical scenario:

A retired businessman and his spouse have led a comfortable life for a number of years in an adult community in the suburbs of a larger city. They have both noticed that he has begun forgetting words, and both became alarmed when he was found wandering in the parking garage of his building. He had forgotten what floor his apartment was on and could not find his way back. His wife urged him to go to their primary-care physician for an appointment, and she accompanied him. When they arrived in the doctor's office, the doctor listened to his patient's concerns and gave them a referral to a cognitive clinic near their home. There, he told them, the husband could take a memory test and get more information.

The clinic, small but well designed, is actually tucked away on a neighborhood side street off a busier highway. The couple is welcomed by a receptionist sitting behind a wooden desk. A vase of fresh flowers, colorful framed prints on the wall, and overstuffed wing chairs add to the welcoming feel. After a short wait, the husband and wife are ushered into an examination room. Its layout is typical: desk, chair, and examination table. But sunlight streams through the venetian blinds that slant against a window, and there is a curtain that can be drawn around the table, for privacy. A physician who is comfortable with memory disorders—perhaps a neurologist or a geriatrician, or an internist—introduces herself to her new patient and to his wife, and sits down to listen. The silver-haired husband and his wife, who still carries herself like the varsity tennis player she was in college, seem alert and engaged, if worried. The doctor is engaged, as well. She knows that she has more time to devote to hearing this couple's story than a fifteen-minute office visit would allow.

Although the physician has been trained in the classical medical model, where advice on disease prevention and healthy lifestyles fall outside her purview, she has moved beyond the confines of that limiting standard. She knows that many elderly people have more than one medical condition, a history that a doctor with a two-thousand-patient workload would not be able to probe—no matter what sort of health services she wanted to provide. As she jots down notes about the patient and his complaint about memory loss, she slips in questions about current events. The conversation flows naturally, but it is in fact a guided conversation designed to assess the patient's memory. The doctor asks about family history, social history, and then makes inquiries about organ systems—heart, lungs, stomach, gut, urinary tract. The patient recalls quite a bit about his medical history, but he struggles once or twice to find the right word. His wife, a bit anxious, rushes to fill in the gap.

When the history is complete, the neurologist asks the patient to don a cotton gown, and she leaves the room for a bit to give the couple some privacy. When the doctor returns, she does a physical examination and selects a set of tests to order from the lab: she asks for samples of blood and urine, but decides no x-rays or MRIs or other scans are needed at this point. A neuropsychologist comes in, greets the couple by name, and leads them to an adjoining room, where the man will be given a more formal memory test and a social worker will join them to come up with an immediate plan for action.

That plan will recommend medications currently on the market, which may give a small boost, and nonpharmaceutical interventions. In a more traditional setting, many of these treatments would fall outside the bounds of the current medical model. But in the cognitive shop, all reasonable and safe interventions are discussed and considered by the staff, including dietary adjustments, supplements, lifestyle adjustments, exercise programs, games and puzzles, and other methods used to challenge the brain. But the person who discusses these interventions is not the physician. The cognitive shop has a Navigator, a position that may seem unfamiliar because it is so new. The Navigator works in a room with a comfortable leather couch, and a large flat screen on one wall. She offers the couple a cup of green tea, and then turns on a laptop computer designed to project a simple Google search page on the screen. She does not know everything, of course, but she is not expected to. With the Internet as her aid, all information about memory loss and Alzheimer's disease is available. Her skill is as a human search engine.

The retired businessman and his wife have scores of questions for the Navigator: Is there a support group for spouses nearby? How can I get help cleaning the house? Is there a grocer who delivers? If we change our diets, will it stave off dementia? What about driving? Do our children have some genetic risk of developing the same problem? Are there any clinical trial programs available? What, if anything, should we tell our friends? Our grandchildren? The Navigator clicks on certain Web sites that are chock-full of useful information, on everything from diet to political activism on Alzheimer's disease. The Navigator prints out a packet that is especially tailored for the husband and wife, and has information they can give to their adult children on what to expect, and what help might be needed down the road. Finally, the Navigator enrolls them in an online site that coordinates volunteer "helpers" in their community, and walks them through a form they may need in the future to file an insurance claim for a home health aide. She asks if there is anything else they need; grateful, but slightly overwhelmed, the couple takes the sheaf of information and schedules a series of follow-up appointments. Although the follow-up visits are not with the neurologist, the couple believes they are in good hands with the cognitive shop staff, and knows that a doctor will oversee any medical needs that might arise.

Too good to be true? Not really. Given the fact that Alzheimer's disease is already the nation's third most expensive disease, costing the government more than $100 billion per year, there is every reason to be open to experimentation with new ways of delivering care.[2] And care that involves the entire family, in an easily accessible neighborhood setting, makes sense for a disease that is, at its essence, a family disease. In 2009, the Alzheimer Study Group estimates, 10 million caregivers will provide 94 billion hours of physically demanding, emotionally draining, uncompensated care.[3] Although the cognitive shop may seem financially out of reach, when weighed against current practice, it is more likely to reduce medical costs. The cognitive shop distributes high-quality care to the community rather than concentrating such care at centralized tertiary-care centers, it reduces physician contact time by having a staff on site that are geared to cognitive health issues, it may delay entry to assisted living facilities and prevent visits to the emergency room, it consolidates care around a major problem that is now handled by a highly fragmented system, it addresses the needs and questions of families, and it adds value to the practices of local primary-care physicians. Because not all of the services available in the cognitive shop are reimbursed by public and private health insurance, the cognitive shop uses a network approach to funding: some money comes from private philanthropy, some from grants, and some from insurance. In addition, the shop works with partner organizations in the neighborhood—a university health club, a local dieticians' group, a yoga instructor, and a local computer guru who is an expert in setting up online social networking sites—to supply a network of low-cost services.

Patient-centered movements have pushed the medical establishment before. The hospice movement, as we have noted, restored a level of humanity to the wrenching process of death and dying. Breast cancer patients, a traditionally well-organized, vocal group, demanded alternative treatments to the disfiguring radical mastectomy in the 1970s, and new research blossomed that changed standards. AIDS patients and caregivers adopted tactics from the civil rights movement of the 1960s to bring public attention to the rise of the human immunodeficiency virus (HIV) in the early 1980s. New experiments in delivering primary medical care, such as the "medical house" movement that gathers care together in one setting, offer a pathway toward healthcare reform.

Although many details remain to be worked out, the cognitive shop offers a similar sort of new paradigm for Alzheimer's disease care and, more important, Alzheimer's disease prevention. It draws together, under one roof, three key steps in a multipronged assault on the many cumulative insults that eventually lead to Alzheimer's disease. Each step involves a care team with physicians and lay experts working in concert to keep the needs of patients and families at the forefront:

Step One: Prevention. We now have good evidence for a set of preventive measures, including diet, exercise, and cognitive stimulation, that can be undertaken. If adopted, these interventions can delay the onset of the disease.

Step Two: Early detection. It is essential to detect Alzheimer's disease in the brain before a person becomes impaired. This means using the tools of genomic medicine and twenty-first-century medicine: genetic predictions, biomarker testing, brain imaging, and baseline neuropsychological testing.

Step Three: A personalized approach to a program of early intervention that helps patients, families, and caregivers navigate the thicket of information on the Internet, and make sense of products on the market.

These steps, taken together, will help patients, families, caregivers, and doctors with the burden of an impending demographic explosion in Alzheimer's cases—and establish a culture of guided experimentation that can only inform the twenty-first-century debate about how to deliver healthcare.

NOTES

1. "A National Alzheimer's Strategic Plan: The Report of the Alzheimer's Study Group," p. 5, http://www.alzstudygroup.org (accessed August 8, 2009).

2. Ibid, p. 4.

3. Ibid.

INDEX